The Science Within

A Heathen Warriors Fitness Manual

The Science Within

A Heathen Warriors Fitness Manual

MICHAEL G. WILLIAMS

Bella's Book Press LLC
https://www.bellarayne.com

Other Titles by Michael C. Williams

Supplement to this Manual:
1 Year Calendar Training Journal For
The Science Within A Heathen Warriors Fitness Manual

The Science Within A Heathen Warriors Fitness Manual
Copyright © Michael C. Williams, 2023
Published by Bella's Book Press LLC

ALL RIGHTS RESERVED

This Manual or any portion thereof may not be reproduced by any electronic, digital, mechanical, photographic, or in the form of a phonographic recording, nor shall it be stored in a retrieval system, transmitted or copied for public or private use…other than under "Fair use" as a brief quotation within articles and reviews…without the prior consent of the Author and or Publisher.
Book Art, photos, images, graphs, calendar, W.O.D. art, reference sheets, and Calendar Log journal are all property of Michael C Williams. All Workout protocols contained within this Manual are the creation of the Author.

ISBN-13:979-8-9881217-3-2 (Hardcover)
ISBN-13:979-8-9881217-0-1 (Paperback)
ISBN-13:979-8-9881217-1-8 (eBook)

Library of Congress Control Number: 2023906461

Special Fonts through Free use with a Commercial License
https://www.1001fonts.com/
Canva pro was used to assist in creating the Book Cover
https://www.canva.com

Disclaimer

The information provided in this Manual was created to provide helpful information on the subjects discussed both Educationally and Informatively. This Manual is not meant to be used, nor should it be used to diagnose or treat any medical condition. There is no implied or expressed guarantee of results should you follow the trainings included in this Manual.
The publisher and author are not responsible for any specific health or allergy requirements for medical supervision. They are not liable for any damages or negative consequences from any treatment, action, application, or preparation to any person reading, applying, or following the information in this Manual.
I recommend consulting a doctor or family physician to assess any health-related issues before dramatically changing your diet or exercise lifestyle.

Bella's Book Press LLC
2184 Channing Way #325
Idaho Falls, Idaho 83404
https://www.bellarayne.com/
https://www.bellarayne.com/heathen-warrior

Dedication

To my family and friends: Please accept my sincere gratitude for all the love and support you have shown me over the years. **You know who you are**. A special thanks to my dear sister T.D.B. Had it not been for your support, this fitness Manual would not have found its way into the world for whoever is reading it. Thank you, NJ, for all your help.

In loving memory of my Dad and Mom and brother Thad. I know you would all be proud of this creation. R.I.P.

Shout out to Tristin and Quintin. I wish you all the best, and I love you both.

Warrior cheers to all the badass women and men competing at the CrossFit Games and Spartan O.C.R. You're amazing! Also, I would like to thank all the athletes out there entertaining the world.

Thank you!

Table of Contents

Introduction

Free the Mind, Challenge the Body, and Educate yourself. You will soon discover, as I did, that Fitness Exercise Sciences are relatively straightforward once you familiarize yourself with the relationship shared among the most common Exercise Physiological terms. If you are engineering a Fitness Program based on Applied Available Science and mathematical formulas or following an Exercise Program, you have all the tools to reach your fitness levels and educational goals. Apply those tools…Achievements will come!

Why I Wrote this Fitness Manual!

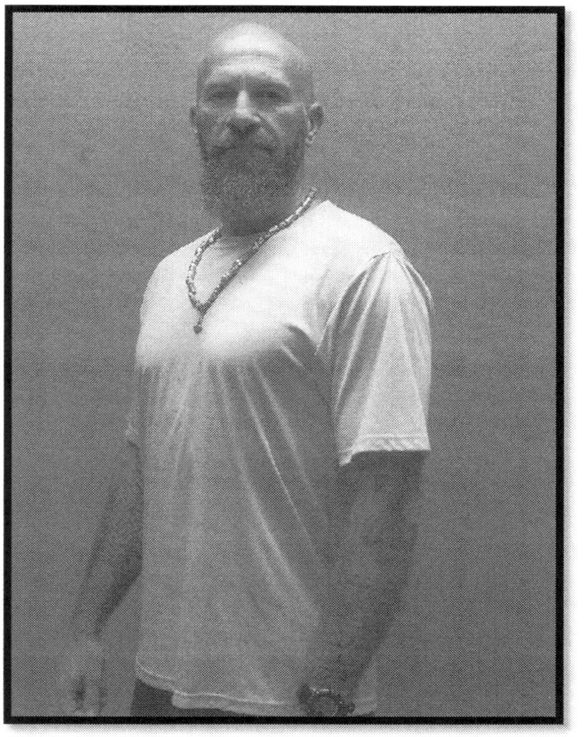

One moment in time, I was a Dad raising two incredible sons while chasing a career in Nuclear engineering. And the next moment, I am an inmate running marathons around a prison yard…WTF…Right?

Life can and will throw us all curve balls. Well, I caught my curve ball on April 6, 2006. This was the day I began a twenty-five-year sentence in prison. The sentence offered minimal shock after watching the entire judicially flawed and corrupted railroad lay tracks straight through my self-defense trial. I hit the prison yard at thirty-two with a twenty-five-year mountain of time ahead of me. Currently, as I write this, now forty-nine years old and almost seventeen years later, I am looking down the other side of that mountain of time with a short eight-year downhill hike to the Gates of Freedom (2031)

When I reflect on the last seventeen years while imprisoned, the time has not been wasted. On the contrary, I have accomplished many things within these walls that I would not have likely pursued as a free younger man chasing a career. Among the many accomplishments has undoubtedly been the Education in Exercise Physiology. It set the tone for redirecting my Sense of Purpose in challenging Both MIND and BODY. Fast forward to February 2014, near my 41st birthday, the prison recreation department announced that they would facilitate the first-ever sanctioned 13.1-mile half-marathon race in April of that year, giving potential participants roughly six to eight weeks to prepare.

You will discover so much about yourself while training for your first half-marathon in prison. The recreation schedule outdoors is inconsistent at times. Security lockdowns or severe weather conditions could interrupt training progress on any given day or week. I won that first half-marathon race in 1:35.19 on April 5, 2014. Out of 2000 plus individuals, only four of us started and finished that race. I still have the group photo. Sharing that training and race experience with three other new runners is definitely among my favorite accomplishments, and it made me HUNGRY for more.

In 2015 I accepted a job transfer from the dog training program to work in the recreation department. From 2015 to 2018, I successfully defended the half marathon title a dozen times. As other events became available, I set facility records in the 5-kilometer, 10-kilometer, and 50-kilometer races. When I departed that facility in June 2018, I was undefeated in all the cross-strength Exercise event competitions.

Not only did I train for my first 26.2-mile marathon…I won it six consecutive times. The Apex of my running achievements is the pair of 50-kilometer ultra-marathons I participated in. Plus, making history by being the first medium custody inmate to do so.

While working in the recreation department, I began redirecting my energy to collaborating with new runners seeking a positive outlet while serving their prison sentences. In addition, teaching what I've learned through course study and applying Exercise Science personally regarding the psychological, mental, and physical fitness health benefits have given my time in prison a sense of purpose and direction.

A famous prison quote, "Do the time or the time will do you!" This quote speaks to every free soul living in the real world or imprisoned. There are positive folks everywhere making the most of life. But, of course, there will always be negative-minded people that are miserable and constantly seeking others to share that misery with. I have chosen to make the most of this current circumstance in the most positive and productive way possible.

Free the Mind, Challenge the Body, Educate Yourself, and you will discover as I did that Fitness Exercise Sciences are relatively straightforward once you familiarize yourself with the relationship shared among the most common Exercise physiological terms. Whether you are engineering a fitness program based on the applied Available Science and mathematical formulas or following a program, YOU possess all the TOOLS in reaching individual fitness or educational goals; use those tools, and achievements will come.

TO EVERYBODY READING THIS

Do the time, Walk Tall, Keep your chin up, Stay focused, and Work Hard.

If we fail to share knowledge from the interpretations of our education and lessons learned, we are part of the problem. That is why I wrote this Fitness Manual! Always remember that Physical Fitness and Mental Health are both equally important. Find Symmetrical Balance within the VOID.
Heathen Warrior

Anaerobic Vo2/Cross-Exercise

Muscular Endurance

Max Cardio And

Recovery Interval Training

For Everybody!

Whether you are a Soldier in the Military fighting for the country, a First Responder risking his/her life for the community, Construction Worker, Truck Driver, Warehouse Worker, Blue Collar, White Collar, or an Inmate wearing prison blues, The Science Within A Heathen Warriors Fitness Manual can be aligned with anybody's lifestyle or daily/weekly Exercise routines.

Whether the work shift begins at 12 a.m. or 6 a.m., you will either be that person running late for work, missing breakfast completely, or the routine for breakfast is a coffee with a bagel. So here are a couple of things to keep in mind.

My family sent me an online prison food gift package for my birthday. A dozen cinnamon raisin bagels were among the variety of food items. For breakfast/pre-exercise meal, I ate a bagel with a cup of coffee for twelve days. I discovered that the nutritional contents of the bagels were adequate for fueling my body through one-hour Exercise routines, low to max intensity levels Av^2/ceme-mc and rit, Fast tempo 5 kilometers, or slow tempo 10-kilometer runs.

The carbohydrates contained within this Cinnamon Raisin bagel is my primary focus. This is Fuel to recharge my Glycogen levels pre-Exercise.

****Low Dietary Fiber @ 3 grams means very little chance of experiencing gastrointestinal distress (Diarrhea) during intense training****

***Note:** Generic prison bagels with peanut butter and jelly contain enough calories to power a body through a one-hour exercise routine. Similar brands of bagels and condiments are available at any supermarket.

This is an example of managing pre-workout calorie intake for specific training only and based on individual needs. Consult a physician before consuming anything new, as there may be food allergy concerns! *

For all the folks getting up every day to chase those careers with very little time to enjoy breakfast at home or finding the time for a gym membership, here are alternatives for maintaining a Fitness level wherever that office is.

Keep in mind that the Science of Fitness is simple. Elevate your Heart Rate to 70-80% of Max, Recover, Repeat, Burn Calories, and build strength and Endurance: See the reference chart in Section 4, Calculating Effort Intensity /Calorie Expense.

2x-Av^2/ci equals two intervals total time at 7.30.00. Perform this routine three times daily and as many times throughout the day as possible. The Goal is 75 to 100 minutes per week.

Perform two intervals of Av^2/ci (Cross Exercises) intermittently throughout the day…the time and Calorie expense will add up. Percentage of Heart Rate Max dictates Calorie expense: 75% for a 180-pound man's Calorie expense at an estimated 73.75 Calories in 7.5 minutes.

See Chart

Choose Exercises that fit your work area surroundings:

Example of Exercises:

Burpees	Push-ups
Vertical Bicycle Crunches	Body Squats
Lunges	Jumping Jacks
Sit-ups	Mountain Climbers

Objective: Elevate your Heart Rate at the office, when possible, during the day without breaking into an uncomfortable sweat at work.

Heads Up:

This is NOT the Gym or your Home. Please DO NOT assume that the Author or the Publisher promotes Poor Work Ethics!

Take

A

Knee

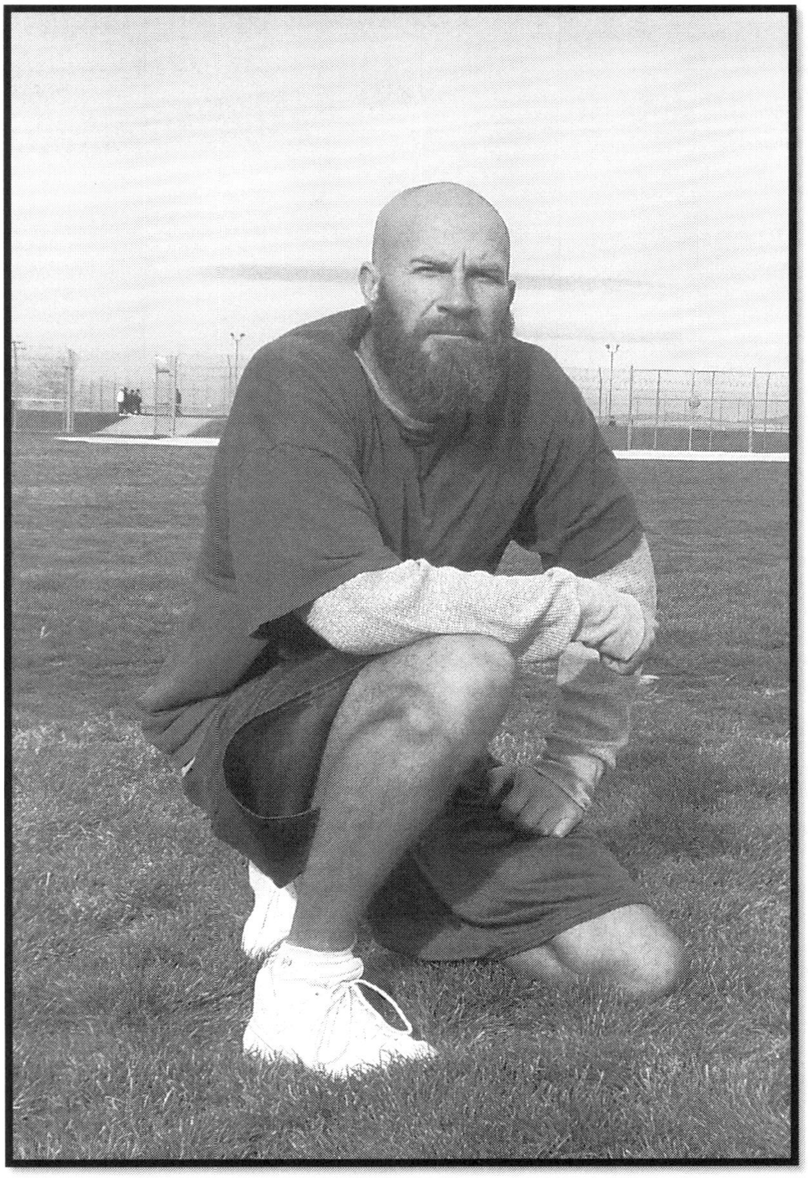

There are precautions to consider when exercising at maximum effort in excessive indoor/outdoor temperatures outside normal training scenarios:
Temperatures 10° to 30° Higher than normal
Outdoor competitions during the Summer months
(M.I.I.T.) Maximum Intensity Interval Training
New to Max effort training
You are still acclimating to higher temperatures
Before you begin an exercise routine in excessive temperatures, ask yourself these questions:
Am I physically prepared to execute this Exercise challenge safely?
Am I hydrated/dehydrated?
Do I have enough fuel for the Exercise routine?
During the Exercise challenge, evaluate yourself in case you need to deviate to address the following:

Overheated	**Feeling Vertigo (Dizzy)**
Tunnel Vision (Sight)	**Body Chills**
Tips of Extremities Tingle	**Cramping**
Heart Rate Management	**Breathing Management Erratic**
Nausea	**Vomiting**

***Note**

If you are feeling vertigo, temporarily abort the Exercise. Take a knee and breathe. Taking a knee places you closer to the ground in case of a fall or fainting…Less chance of a severe head injury event.*

Re-establishing a lower Heart Rate and Breathing may only take seconds for recovery. In more severe cases where the conditions are extremely Hot or Humid, more than 90° to 100° +/-, it may take minutes for your core temperature to drop enough to resume the Exercise routine safely; Assess your risks versus rewards in continuing. If you decide to cease the Exercise routine Challenge or Competition, never accept this circumstance as a failure or mistake. Instead, use it as a learning experience tool to use next time. Remember, there is always tomorrow or next week. But there is no tomorrow or next week if you injure yourself physically or mentally and bruise your self-confidence.
Final notes on this subject for redundancy.
Do not stumble around Gym equipment when feeling Vertigo.
Take a Knee and Execute the Following Steps:

1	**Breathe**
2	**Compose Yourself**
3	**Focus**

Assess the situation and check your Heart Rate to be sure it is within a normal range.

When it comes to safety, knowing one's own normal or familiar heart rate is important This initial Heart Rate will give you so much information. Check it every 30 to 40 seconds until it has dropped 12 to 24 beats per minute.
Take a Breath and Stand up slowly. Then, if you still feel Vertigo, "Take a knee and Repeat these steps until you can stand up safely.
Again, these recovery steps only take seconds. When you feel confident in continuing the Exercise…

"EMBRACE MORE SUCK"

OR

"SAVE YOURSELF FOR ANOTHER DAY!"

Tempo = Intensity

Tempo in Hot, humid conditions = Intensity^2

Temperature-related training and competition performance decline above the ideal temperature of 50° Running/Cross Exercise Training:

Expect slower per mile Running and slower per 10 minutes Cross Exercise Training.

@60° 5 seconds slower
@70° 10 seconds slower
@80° 20 seconds slower
@90° 21-40 seconds slower
Temperatures above 90° or humidity levels 40-80% expect a higher rate of performance decline.

Example:

RUNNERS:

Expect performance declines when running from a Max Effort of a 7 minute per mile pace finish time in 50° temperatures running a Max Effort of 7.40.00 to 8 minute per mile pace time in 90° temperatures and humidity levels that exceed 50 to 90% plus/minus.

CROSS-EXERCISE TRAINING ATHLETES:

During Max Effort Cross Exercise Efficiency Training in cool or hot/humid conditions, expect similar performance declines. For example, a Max Effort Workout Interval that takes 10 minutes to complete at a 50° temperature may take 11 minutes to complete at a 90° temperature and when humidity levels exceed 50 to 90% +/-.

Calorie God

or

Calorie Devil

The Magical Number 3500 KCal

3500 Calories: Equals an estimated one pound of body weight via Calorie expenditure living, individual lifestyle, and physical activity. Keep this number in mind as you learn the Science Applied to Fitness and Exercise within this Heathen Warriors Manual…**Which is now your MANUAL!**

Accepting the Calorie God OR not is strictly the reader's decision. However, before you disregard its existence in your life, let me share why the Calorie God is Sustenance for Life, Power, and Achieving Fitness Goals is essential.

Like water and air, we also need Calories to sustain our lives. Without the Calorie God, we cease to be alive, plain and simple. However, decline to bow down in submission. Instead, conclude that, in its simplest form, a Calorie is "Just Fuel." Fuel to live, Fuel to run, and Exercise and Fuel to have fun.

Knowing the Individual Twenty-four-hour total Calorie intake needs can be calculated in Section (2) of this Manual, "How to Calculate Resting Metabolic Rate." Also, knowing how many Calories you need will make managing Calorie expenses through Exercise much more Efficient.

Remember this Analogy:

When filling up a vehicle's gasoline tank, you can pump a certain amount into it before it spills out all over the ground. "Gasoline all over the ground is a waste of fuel, and money, and It Is Dangerous!"

Now you know your daily Calorie intake needs. Consuming more calories than needed will begin to spill over as potentially dangerous unwanted fat storage. "A Body can only Process so much calorie intake before it becomes a Waste of Fuel and Money!"

Now that we are Learning more about Understanding the Importance of Calories let's dive into Applying the Science and Math of Individual Calorie intake based on physiological needs through Self-assessment of Daily/Weekly Physical Activities and Lifestyle. A complete understanding of "CALORIES OUT (vs) CALORIES IN" will help you manage daily intake and balance between becoming Calorie Deficit or consuming more calories than needed. Awareness of the Calories In/Out, whether Consumed or Expended, builds Confidence in the Management Discipline of Daily Calorie Intake and Calorie Expense when Exercising.

It is easier said than done, for sure! But remember, you have the Power of Knowledge. Do not allow the Calorie God to intimidate you. See the Calorie God for what it truly is… "Fuel for Life."

Let's all agree that eating Calories makes us feel good. Here is my philosophy on Eating out of Necessity or Indulgence. I never feel guilty about eating a treat if it makes me feel good or if I believe it has been earned. I eat the treat with complete awareness that it comes with the Calories Out cost in Exercise.

Teach yourself at a glance to understand the Nutritional Facts of any food or drink. Pay close attention to serving size and total Calories per serving. The Calories Out cost for any Indulgence is to pay back with Minutes and Miles of Cross Exercise Training, Rowing, Cycling, Swimming, Running, or Walking. "The Science Within A Heathen Warriors Fitness Manual" is packed with all the management tools needed to learn how to Efficiently Pay the Cost for Calories Consumed.

Here are a few simple miscellaneous Calorie Expense Exercise formulas for Management Data that will give YOU power over the Calorie God and the Calorie Devil:

Refer to Section 4 in this Manual for Calculating Effort Intensity, Performance Level Percentages, and Calorie Expense

Total Body Cardio Strength Interval Training (WR-10) With Run-10 (Cross Exercise Training)
Total Body Cardio Strength Interval Training (NR-10.8) No Run-10.8 (Cross Exercise Training)

CALORIES OUT

Apply these quick formulas for Calorie Expense when Performing the following Exercises:

Running

Multiply the Numbers below by Bodyweight (Pounds) for Calorie Expense per Mile.

Max Tempo Effort Intensity

Zone 1	**@ .735**	**x**	**Bodyweight (Pounds)**	**=**
Zone 2	**@.71**	**x**	**Bodyweight (Pounds**	**=**
Zone 3	**@.685**	**x**	**Bodyweight (Pounds)**	**=**

High Tempo Effort Intensity

Zone 1	**@ .66**	**x**	**Bodyweight (Pounds)**	**=**
Zone 2	**@ .635**	**x**	**Bodyweight (Pounds)**	**=**
Zone 3	**@.61**	**x**	**Bodyweight (Pounds)**	**=**

Low Tempo Effort Intensity

Zone 1	**@.585**	**x**	**Bodyweight (Pounds**	**=**
Zone 2	**@ .56**	**x**	**Bodyweight (Pounds)**	**=**
Zone 3	**@.535**	**x**	**Bodyweight (Pounds)**	**=**

Walking

Low Tempo Effort Intensity

Zone 1	**@.53**	**x**	**Bodyweight (Pounds)**	**=**

"Notice how Tempo, Effort Intensity, and Duration Effects Calorie Expenses."

"Please note, Performing 10 minutes of Cross Exercise Training equals One Mile of Running Economy Dependent upon Tempo and Effort Intensity."

In my experience, paying for a treat is easier than feeling guilty for eating it. And guilt can create a negative domino effect that manifests as misplaced Self-guilt into anxiety and depression… Hence the dreaded "Calorie Devil."

Giving power to the Calorie Devil makes for a highly counterproductive scenario. Therefore, losing focus on achieving our individual goals. Move forward with positive momentum, knowledge, awareness, and discipline. If you fail to meet a goal, do not perceive it as a failure or loss. Instead, interpret it as a Learning Experience, Acknowledge the Valuable Lesson, Let it Fuel you, and Continue with a New Goal.

Heathen Warrior Fitness Creed

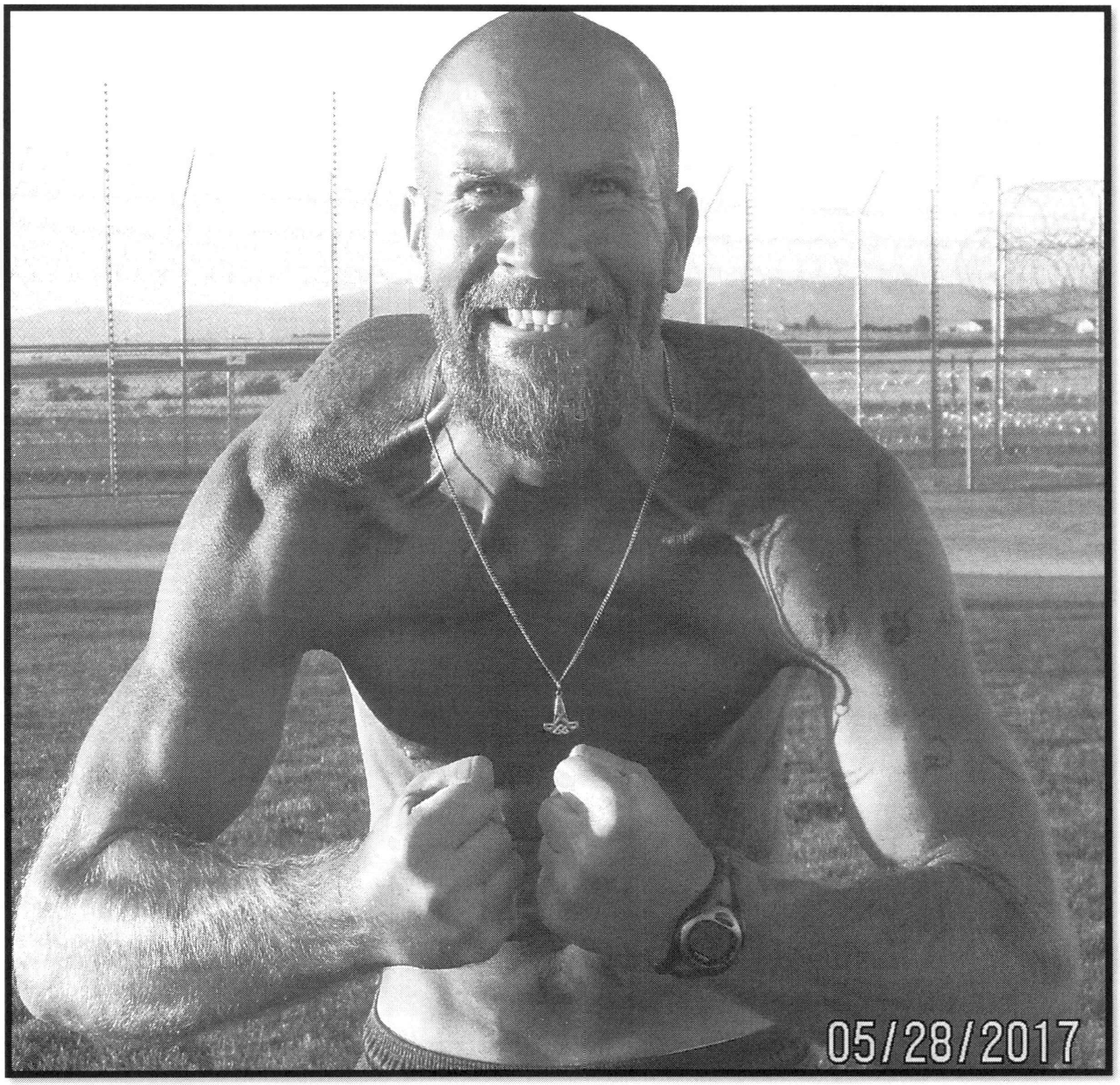

Heathen Warrior Fitness Creed

Lo There, Do I see the EVOLUTION of my
Fitness and Health
Lo There, Do I embrace the WISDOM, and
Spirit of a Raven
Lo There, Do I possess the HEART of a Viking Warrior
charging across the Battlefield at
enemies of old
Lo There, Do I find the STRENGTH in Myself to Complete
Today's Challenges
Lo There, Do I find the ENDURANCE of Wolves
in my Soul
Lo There, Do I SENSE the Suffering of Agony
and Misery as Weakness Leaving my Body
Lo There, Do I HONOR the Ancient Souls of
Norsemen Folk celebrating in the
Halls of Valhalla
Lo, I am Heathen Reigned!

Section 1:

Body Composition

Metrication

Body Composition Metrication

Metric Conversion is a simple process of mathematical steps. Follow the steps in this section for the Metric Conversions of an individual's body weight and height.

Please note
Unless your Body Composition changes significantly, continue to use your Conversion Number(s) for the Metric Formulas in this Manual.

Step One:
Body Mass (Weight) (_____) Pounds ÷ by 2.2046 =
Body Mass (Weight) (_____) Kilograms (kg)

Step Two:
Stature (Height) (____) Inches x by 2.54 =
Stature (Height) (____) Centimeters (cm)

Example for Converting Stature (_____) centimeters to meters and meters squared (M^2)

Stature (Height) (75") inches x by 2.54 equals
Statue (Height) (190.5) centimeters (cm)
190.5 cm ÷ by 100 = (1.905) meters
(1.905 x 1.905) = 3.629 meters Squared (M^2)

Formula Reference:

Current Metricated Body Composition
Body Mass/Weight____________ kilograms (kg)
Stature/Height__________ centimeters (cm)

"*F.Y.I. 2.2046 kilograms equals 1 pound, and 2.54 centimeters equals 1 inch. *"

Section 2:

How to Calculate

Resting Metabolic Rate

Calculate with Energy Expenditure for 24-hour Calorie intake need estimate using the following:

Individual Body Composition Metrication

Body Mass_________ Kilograms (kg)
Stature_____________ Centimeters (cm)
Current Age________

Multiply the Percentage Value Number assigned that Represents Individual Physical Activity, Exercise Effort Intensity Levels of Training during the Week (1 to 7 Days), and Career (IE) Professional Athlete self-assessment for Total Caloric Need.

Enter your Body Mass (Kilograms) in Designated Slot (A):
Enter your Stature (Centimeters) in Designated Slot (B)
Enter your Age (Years) in Designated Slot (C)

A	**Weight (kg)**	x 10	= slot (a)_____
B	**Height (cm)**	x 6.25	= slot (b)_____
C	**Age**	x 5 + 5	= slot (c)_____

slot A + slot B – slot C =_______ x Self-Assessment Value Number =______Total Calories Needed Per Day (KCal/24 HR)

Self-Assessment:

1.21% **Injury Recovery, Level Three Low-Intensity Exercises, Sedentary, Non-Active Career or Lifestyle**

1.38% **Travel/Vacation, 2 to 4 Low-Intensity Erratic Exercise Days, Moderately Active Career and Lifestyle**

1.56% **5 Day Exercise Schedule Performing Level Two High-Intensity Zones 1 & 2 with Bonus Exercise Days, Very Active Career and Lifestyle**

1.73% **7 Day Exercises at Level One Max Intensity Zone 2 and Level Two High-Intensity Zones 1 & 2, Advanced Competitive Level Training, High Energy Lifestyle, and Very Active Career**

1.91% **7 Day Exercises at Level One Max Intensity Zones 1 & 2, advanced Competitive level Training at Maximum Effort Intensity Heart Rate Zones, Physically Active Career, and High Energy Lifestyle**

Example:

(A) Weight (kg) 81.65 x 10 = 816.50 = (A)
(B) Height (cm) 190.5 x 6.25 = 1190.6 = (B)
(C)Age 35 x 5 + 5 = 180 = (C)
(A + B – C=) 816.50 + 1190.6 – 180 = 1827.1
Final Step: Multiply 1827.1 by Self-assessment value 1.73% = 3160.9 KCal/24 HR

Section 3:

Body Mass

Index (BMI)

*Please note that the Science is not always accurate for Individual **BMI Scores** as there exists a broad range of Body Composition types; athletic and non-athletic. *

Body Mass Index (BMI)

First BMI formula

Follow the steps in the example and then get your calculator ready for entering individual data.

Example:

Body Weight is in pounds, and Height is inches squared
***For example: (inches x inches) ***

Weight (Pounds)	÷ by	Height inches squared	x by	= Score
140	÷ by	(67" x 67") =4489	x by	705 = _____Score

(BMI = 140 ÷ 4489 x 705= 21.99 Score)

Enter Individual Data for Estimated BMI

Bodyweight _____pounds ÷ By Height (inches x inches) = ______x by 705 =

(BMI = _____ ÷ _____ x 705 = _____ Score)

Second Opinion BMI Formula

Bodyweight is in kilograms and Height is in meters^2 *For Example: (meters x meters) *
Weight ______(kg) ÷ by Height (meters^2) _______= BMI Score________ (kg ÷ M^2)
Formula Breakdown

Example:

Weight	**140 Pounds**	**÷ by**	**2.2046**	**=**	**63.50 (kg)**
Height	**67 inches**	**x by**	**2.54**	**=**	**170.18 (cm)**
Height	**170.18 (cm)**	**÷ by**	**100**	**=**	**1.7018 meters**
Height	**1.7018 meters**	**x by**	**1.7018 meters**	**=**	**2.896 (M^2)**

BMI = 63.50 (kg) ÷ 2.896 (M^2) = 21.92 Score *(kg ÷ M^2) *

Body Mass Index Scale
Estimated Ideal Health Range Score: 18.5 to 24.9
Estimated Low to Moderate health Risk Score: 0 to 18.4
Estimated Moderate to Elevated Health Risk Score: 25 to 40

Section 4:

Calculating Effort Intensity, Performance Level Percentages, & Calorie Expense Per Minute for WR-10 and NR-10.8 training only!

For Calculating Effort Intensity, Performance Level Percentages, and Calorie Expense Per Minute for WR-10 and NR-10.8 training only!

Total Body Cardio Strength Interval Training (WR-10) With Run-10
Total Body Cardio Strength Interval Training (NR-10.8) No Run-10.8

Total body Cardio Strength Interval Training **With Run (or) No Run** can be performed with/without recovery between exercises unless following a specific routine. Otherwise, it is at the discretion of the individual to choose the order of how each Exercise is executed.
In this section, you will find significant differences between these training types, **WR-10 and NR-10.8**. Please familiarize yourself with the difference before you begin any calculations. The numbers have been assigned to each training type to Represent a Variable for accurate KCal per minute Data Estimate.

Description of each training type with number variable

Total body Cardio Strength Interval Training **(WR-10)**
With Run-10 (WR-10) *1 kilometer + Running required for KCal accuracy* Example: How this Variable is Applied in the calculation.
KCal Value x body weight (pounds) ÷ 10 (WR) = KCal Per Minute
Total Body Cardio Strength Interval Training **(NR-10.8)**
No Run10.8 (NR-10.8)

Example: How this Variable is Applied in the Calculation

KCal Value x Body weight (Pounds) ÷ 10.8 (NR) = KCal Per Minute

Practice these calculations using the examples for both training types on the following page. Then practice applying your body composition information until you are confident applying all the training data in the calculation process.
Practice taking your 10-second Heart Rate Pulse. It is extremely important. The best location to find a strong and consistent pulse is inside the point where your left collarbone meets the neck. The Subclavian Artery works well as it is close to the heart.
10-second pulse rate multiplied by ten equals (BPM) Beats Per Minute
Feel free to use the Heart Rate monitor in quality fitness watches or chest strap monitors. Follow device instructions for the best accuracy. Test this device against an actual pulse rate for consistency.

The information on this page will show the significant differences in total Calorie expense between the following two aforementioned:

Total Body Cardio Interval Training WR-10) With Run-10
Total Body Cardio Strength Interval Training (NR-10.8) No Run-10.8

These Examples below will instruct the Calculation Process and how to use the calculation chart on page three of this Section.

Please note the following for your practice calculations
Apply the same workout duration for both examples (45 minutes)
Apply the same average Heart Rate (171 BPM) for both examples
Differences to be aware of: Female, Male, Bodyweight (Pounds), and Age-related Formulas for Heart Rate Max (HrMx) via advanced versus nonadvanced Cardio experience with Run and No Run Scenarios.

1st Scenario

Hella is 35 years old, bodyweight at 145 pounds, and considers herself with Advanced Cardio Experience.
Use the following (HrMx) Formula, (211 - 64 x Age 35) = 188.6 BPM (HrMx)
Hella completed a 5km Run and Total Body Strength Training Intervals in 45 minutes with an average Heart Rate of 171 BPM (171 ÷ 188.6 = 90%)
***Find 90% and KCal value on the chart* 90% = Level 2 High-Intensity Effort Zone One: KCal Value (.74)**

Calculation

.74 x Bodyweight (145 pounds) ÷ by With Run-10 = 10.73 KCal Per Minute

10.73 KCal Per Minute x 45-minute Total Training Duration = 482.85 CALORIE EXPENSE

2nd Scenario

Thor is 21 years old. Body weight at 165 pounds and considers himself a Non-advanced Cardio Experience
Use the following HrMx Formula 220 – Age (21) = 199 BPM HrMx
Thor completed a 45-minute Total body Cardio Strength Training Routine with an Average Heart Rate of 171 BPM (171 ÷ 199= 86%)
***Find 86% and KCal Value on Chart* 86% = Level Two High-Intensity Effort Zone One: KCal Value (.70)**

Calculation

.70 x Bodyweight (165 Pounds) ÷ No Run-10.8 = 10.69 KCal Per Minute

10.69 KCal Per Minute x 45-minute Total Training Duration = 481.25 CALORIE EXPENSE

Tempo equals intensity

Adding a significant portion of running to your Total Body Interval Training requires a higher Calorie expense, as expressed within the calculation charts' effort intensity: (levels and zones).

See Section (4) for Practice Breaking down (A.L.O.I.) Average Level of Intensity

Calculation chart for finding your Effort Intensity Level Zone with an assigned value number for calculating Calorie expense when performing or competing in **Total Body Interval Training challenges**.

Use the chart below to locate your Effort Intensity using the correlating percentage of your Heart Rate Max from the average beats per minute data log during Total Body workouts. Then calculate Calorie expense with the value number provided for all three training levels and zones:

Level One % of HrMx =		Maximum Intensity Effort Intensity	
Zone One		**Zone Two**	
100%	**.84 KCal Value**	**95%**	**.79 KCal Value**
99%	**.83 KCal Value**	**94%**	**.78 KCal Value**
98%	**.82 KCal Value**	**93%**	**.77 KCal Value**
97%	**.81 KCal Value**	**92%**	**.76 KCal Value**
96%	**.80 KCal Value**	**91%**	**.75 KCal Value**

Level Two % of HrMx =				High Intensity Effort Intensity	
Zone One		**Zone Two**		**Zone Three**	
90%	**.74 KCal Value**	**85%**	**.69 KCal Value**	**80%**	**.64 KCal Value**
89%	**.73 KCal Value**	**84%**	**.68 KCal Value**	**79%**	**.63 KCal Value**
88%	**.72 KCal Value**	**83%**	**.67 KCal Value**	**78%**	**.62 KCal Value**
87%	**.71 KCal Value**	**82%**	**.66 KCal Value**	**77%**	**.61 KCal Value**
86%	**.70 KCal Value**	**81%**	**.65 KCal Value**	**76%**	**.60 KCal Value**

Level Three	Low Intensity
% of HrMx =	Effort Intensity

Zone One		Zone Two		Zone Three	
75%	.59 KCal Value	70%	.54 KCal Value	65%	.49 KCal Value
74%	.58 KCal Value	69%	.53 KCal Value	64%	.48 KCal Value
73%	.57 KCal Value	68%	.52 KCal Value	63%	.47 KCal Value
72%	.56 KCal Value	67%	.51 KCal Value	62%	.46 KCal Value
71%	.55 KCal Value	66%	.50 KCal Value	61%	.45 KCal Value

Section 5:

Running

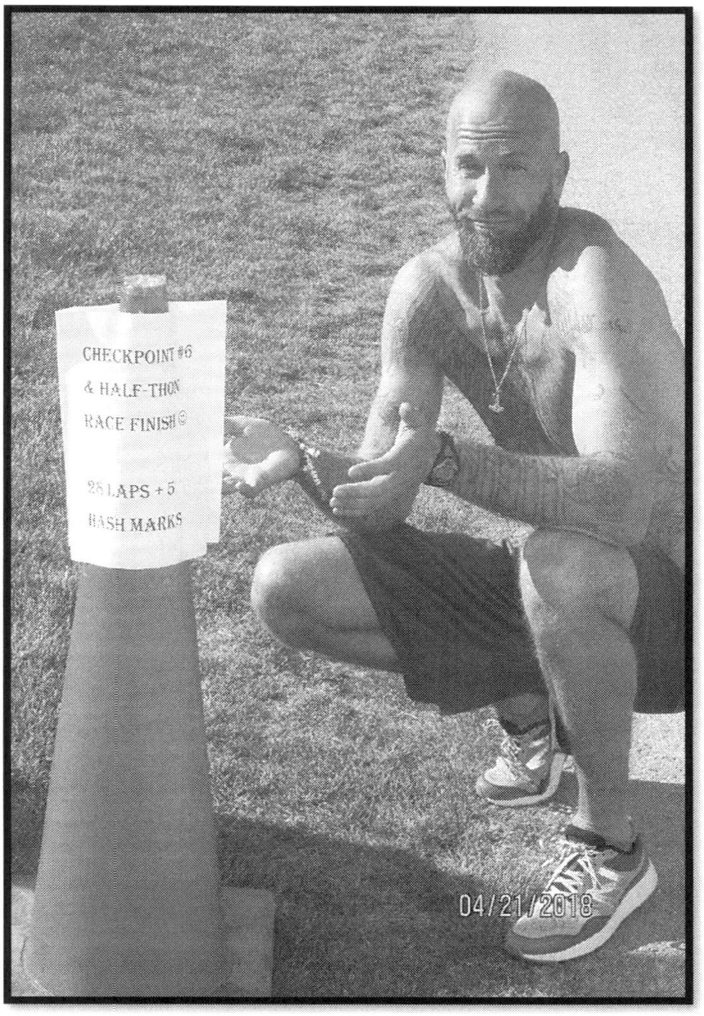

- **FOR RUNNING ONLY**
  The chart to Find Tempo Effort Intensity Percentage
- 5k & 10k
  6-Week Training Plan(s)
- TwQ 6 x 10^3 Algorithm Time Key Chart
- 6 x 10^3 = 6,000 (1/100ths) = (One Minute TwQ Algorithm Key) mcw '13-22
- 1 kilometer PR @100% Effort Intensity/Training Percentage Zones
- Goal Pace Key for Estimated Finish Times
- Average Level of Intensity (A.L.O.I.) & Percentage of Physical Output (P.O.P.O.)

FOR RUNNING ONLY

Use the chart to find the Tempo Effort Intensity Percentage of Individual Heart Rate Max from Post Run Exercise Data. Then calculate Calorie Expense with the **KCal Value** number assigned to all three levels and nine zones.

Level One
Max Tempo Effort Intensity

Zone 1	Zone 2	Zone 3
100% KCal Value .735	95% KCal Value .71	90% KCal Value .685
99% KCal Value .73	94% KCal Value .705	89% KCal Value .68
98% KCal Value .725	93% KCal Value .70	88% KCal Value .675
97% KCal Value .72	92% KCal Value .695	87% KCal Value .67
96% KCal Value .715	91% KCal Value .69	86% KCal Value .665

Level Two
High Tempo Effort Intensity

Zone 1	Zone 2	Zone 3
85% KCal Value .66	80% KCal Value .635	75% KCal Value .61
84% KCal Value .655	79% KCal Value .63	74% KCal Value .605
83% KCal Value .65	78% KCal Value .625	73% KCal Value .60
82% KCal Value .645	77% KCal Value .62	72% KCal Value .595
81% KCal Value .64	76% KCal Value .615	71% KCal Value .59

Level Three
Low Tempo Effort Intensity

Zone 1	Zone 2	Zone 3
70% KCal Value .585	65% KCal Value .56	60% KCal Value .535
69% KCal Value .58	64% KCal Value .555	59% KCal Value .53
68% KCal Value .575	63% KCal Value .55	58% KCal Value .525
67% KCal Value .57	62% KCal Value .545	57% KCal Value .52
66% KCal Value .565	61% KCal Value .54	56% KCal Value .515

Note** that the Level 3 Low Tempo Effort Intensity **Zone Three,** 59% KCal value .53, can be used for Walking Tempo Effort and Calorie Expense with the same Individual Heart Rate Max percentage from Post Walk Exercise Data as above. ***See chart.

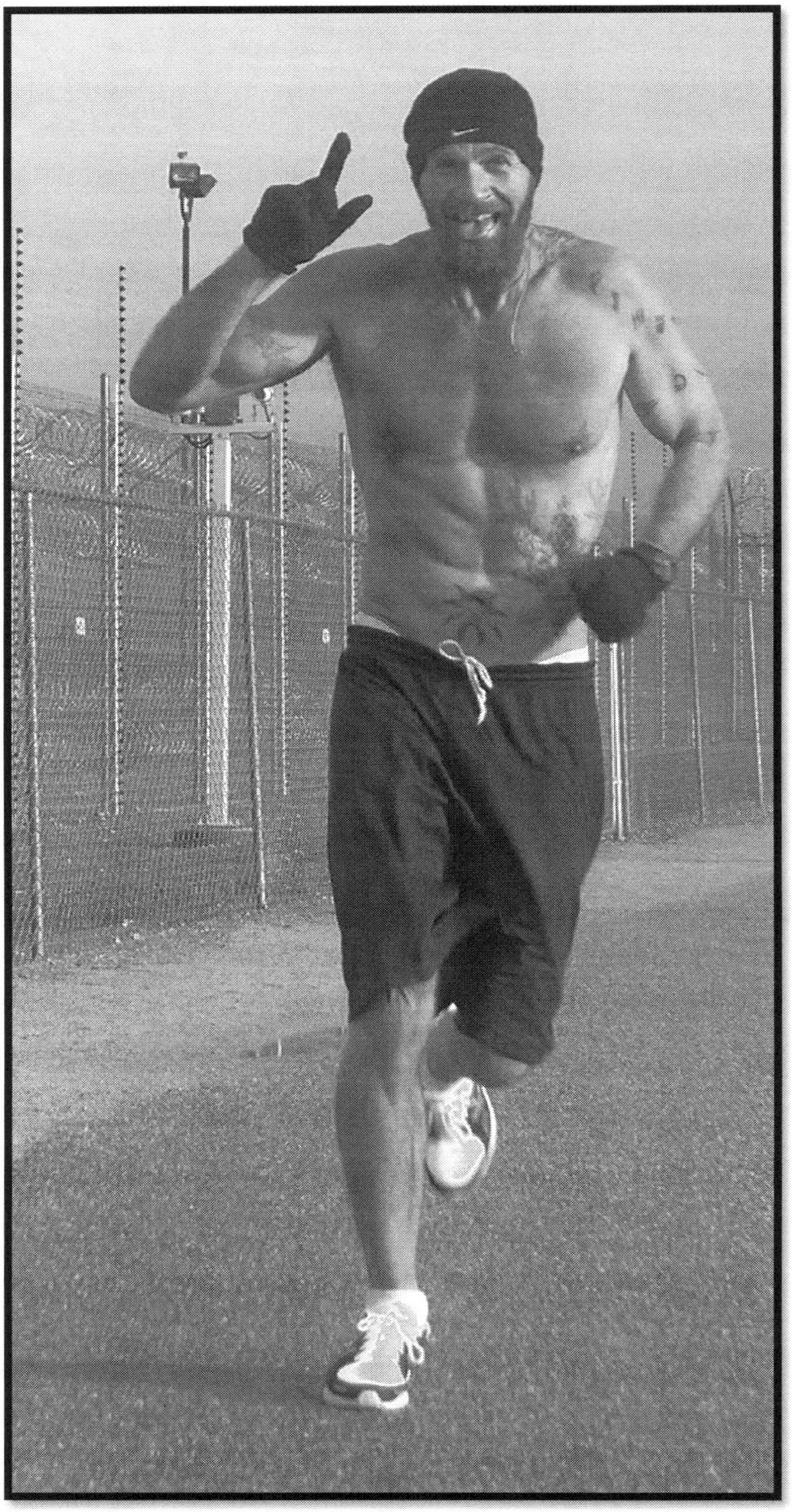

5k & 10k 6-WEEK TRAINING PLANS
42 days to Race Day

First, overlay this plan with an exact goal date for your Run 42 days out for a complete training camp, **or** an improvised training period for experienced runners that do not require a full Six weeks may begin at the training week number that complements the individual needs.

Example:
If the goal run date for the schedule 5K or 10K is 28 days (4 Weeks) to Race Day, begin at:

Week three

Sunday

Day 15

This provides 28 days of Constructive Training for Race Day Goal
The author of these training plans recommends that inexperienced runners complete the full six weeks of training to reap the best possible results

Refer to Section 5
Goal Pace Key For Estimated Finish Times

Whether you are training for 5K or 10K, the Goal Pace Key in Section 5 is an excellent tool for making a finish time goal. Use the Goal Pace Key chart for setting a presumptive finish time. This table shows the Average kilometer and mile pace necessary for achieving the presumed finish time goal.

See Example: (Information located on the Goal Pace Key chart)

5k Goal Finish Time	**25.50.00**
Average One Kilometer Pace	**5.10.00**
Average One-Mile Pace	**8.18.87**
10k Goal Finish Time	**49.09.97**
Average One Kilometer Pace	**4.55.00**
Average One-Mile Pace	**7.54.73**

Contradiction in Motion

I RUN LIKE CRAZY FOR MY SANITY

Heathen Warrior

Begin the training plan by running 100% Max Effort (Week one). Personal best 1 kilometer (.6214 Miles). This Baseline run will be performed at the beginning of each training week. This Baseline kilometer time is tailored to individual ability and dictates the training pace throughout the week.
Perform the 100% Baseline 1-kilometer time throughout each week, applying the chart data on the **1-kilometer PR @ 100% Effort Intensity/Training Percentage Zones Chart** in Section 5. Become familiar with this chart. It is a necessary tool for the Six Week Plan.

Example:

1 kilometer @ 100% Max Effort Baseline			**Run Time: 4.15.00**		
60% of Baseline (4.15.00)	=	**7.05.00 Per kilometer Pace**	**Total 2k Time Goal**	=	**14.10.00**
75% of Baseline (4.15.00)	=	**5.40.00 Per kilometer Pace**	**Total 3k Time Goal**	=	**16.20.00**
80% of Baseline (4.15.00)	=	**5.18.75 Per kilometer Pace**	**Total 4k Time Goal**	=	**21.15.00**

If this is your first 5K/10K training plan Or 50th, it is engineered for all skill levels.

Note As progress is made each week of the training plan, finish time goals may change multiple times as you get faster, conditioned, and more confident in the training percentages.

Refer to Section 7 in this Manual for Cross Exercise Threshold training instructions that complement Running Tempo Effort Intensity levels:

Section 7:

Av^2/ci Anaerobic Vo2 Cardio Intervals & Av^2/ci 24-Day Training Plan
Av^2/ceme-mc and rit:
AnaerobicVo2/cross-exercise muscular endurance-max cardio and recovery interval training

Trifecta of Training Thresholds

5k & 10k Six-Week Training Plans Week One & Week Two

Week One	Week Two
Sunday Day 1 1km Run (.6214 miles) Max Effort 100% Baseline 4x-Av^2/ci (Low Intensity) *Cross Exercise Training Optional*	Sunday Day 8 1km Run (.6214 miles) Max Effort 100% Week 2 Baseline Av^2/ci *Cross Exercise Training Optional*
Monday Day 2 2km Run (1.2 miles) 5k Plan 4km Run (2.48 miles) 10k Plan At 60% of the Max Effort Baseline 4x-Av^2/ci (Low intensity) *Cross-exercise Training*	Monday Day 9 2km Run (1.2 miles) 5k Plan 4km Run (2.48 miles) 10k Plan At 70% of the Max Effort Baseline 4x-Av^2/ci (High Intensity) *Cross Exercise Training*
Tuesday Day 3 Run Optional 6x-Av^2/ci (Low Intensity) *Cross Exercise Training*	Tuesday Day 10 Run Optional 6x-Av^2/ci (High Intensity) *Cross Exercise Training*
Wednesday Day 4 2km Run (1.2 miles) 5k Plan 4km Run (2.48 miles) 10k Plan At 70% of Max effort Baseline 4x-Av^2/ci (High Intensity) *Cross Exercise Training*	Wednesday Day 11 2km Run (1.2 miles) 5k Plan 4km Run (2.48 miles) 10k Plan At 80% of Max effort Baseline 6x-Av^2/ci (Low Intensity) *Cross Exercise Training*
Thursday Day 5 3km Run (1.86 miles) 5k Plan 6km Run (3.7 miles) 10k Plan At 65% of the Max Effort Baseline 4x-Av^2/ci (Low Intensity) *Cross Exercise Training*	Thursday Day 12 3km Run (1.86 miles) 5k Plan 6km Run (3.7 miles) 10k Plan At 70% of the Max Effort Baseline 4x-Av^2/ci (Max Intensity) *Cross Exercise Training*
Friday Day 6 Complete Rest Optional *Runner's Discretion*	Friday Day 13 Complete Rest Optional *Runner's Discretion*
Saturday Day 7 4km Run/Walk (2.48 miles) 5k Plan 8km Run/Walk (4.97 miles) 10k Plan At 60-65% of the Max Effort Baseline Av^2/ci *Cross-exercise Training Optional*	Saturday Day 14 4km Run (2.48 miles) 5k Plan 8km Run (4.97 miles) 10k Plan At 65-70% of the Max Effort Baseline Av^2/ci *Cross-exercise Training Optional*

5k & 10k Six-Week Training Plans Week Three & Week Four

Week Three	Week Four
Sunday Day 15 1km Run (.6214 miles) Max Effort 100% Week 3 Baseline Av^2/ci *Cross Exercise Training Optional*	Sunday Day 22 1km Run (.6214 miles) Max Effort 100% Week 4 Baseline Av^2/ci *Cross Exercise Training Optional*
Monday Day 16 3km Run (1.86 miles) 5k Plan 6km Run (3.7 miles) 10k Plan At 75% of the Max Effort Baseline 6x-Av^2/ci (Low Intensity) *Cross Exercise Training*	Monday Day 23 4km Run (2.48 miles) 5k Plan 8km Run (4.97 miles) 10k Plan At 80% of the Max Effort Baseline 6x-Av^2/ci (High Intensity) *Cross Exercise Training*
Tuesday Day 17 Run Optional 8x-Av^2/ci (High Intensity) *Cross Exercise Training*	Tuesday Day 24 Run Optional 8x-Av^2/ci (Max Intensity) *Cross Exercise Training*
Wednesday Day 18 2km Run (1.2 miles) 5k Plan 4km Run (2.48 miles) 10k Plan At 85% of the Max Effort Baseline 4x-Av^2/ci (Max Intensity) *Cross Exercise Training*	Wednesday Day 25 4km Run (2.48 miles) 5k Plan 8km Run (4.97 miles) 10k Plan At 70-75% of the Max Effort Baseline 4x-Av^2/ci (Max Intensity) *Cross Exercise Training*
Thursday Day 19 4km Run (2.48 miles) 5k Plan 8km Run (4.97 miles) 10k Plan At 60-70% of the Max Effort Baseline 6x-Av^2/ci (Max Intensity) *Cross Exercise Training*	Thursday Day 26 3km Run (1.86 miles) 5k Plan 6km Run (3.7 miles) 10k Plan At 65% of the Max Effort Baseline 8x-Av^2/ci (Low Intensity) *Cross Exercise Training*
Friday Day 20 Complete Rest Optional *Runner's Discretion*	Friday Day 27 Complete Rest Optional *Runner's Discretion*
Saturday Day 21 4km Run (2.48 miles) 5k Plan 8km Run (4.97 miles) 10k Plan At 70-75% of the Max Effort Baseline Av^2/ci *Cross Exercise Training Optional*	Saturday Day 28 5km Run/Walk (3.1 miles) 5k Plan 10km Run/Walk (6.2 miles) 10k Plan At 60-80% of the Max Effort Baseline *No Av^2/ci Cross Exercise Training Optional*

5k & 10k
Six-Week
Training Plans
Week Five
&
Week Six

Week Five	Final Week Six
Sunday Day 29 1km Run (.6214 miles) Max effort 100% Week 5 Baseline Av²/ci (Optional) *Cross Exercise Training*	Sunday Day 36 1km Run (.6214 miles) Max effort 100% Week 6 Baseline, Taper Week to Race Day Count-down Av²/ci *Cross Exercise Training Optional*
Monday Day 30 5km Run/Walk (3.1 miles) 5k Plan 10km Run/Walk (6.2 miles) 10k Plan At 60-80% of the Max Effort Baseline 4x-Av²/ci (Low Intensity) *Cross Exercise Training*	Monday Day 37 3km Run (1.86 miles) 5k Plan 6km Run (3.7 miles) 10k Plan At 90% of the Max Effort Baseline 4x-Av²/ci (High Intensity) *Cross Exercise Training*
Tuesday Day 31 Run Optional 6x-Av²/ci (High Intensity) *Cross Exercise Training*	Tuesday Day 38 Run Optional 6x-Av²/ci (Low Intensity) *Cross Exercise Training*
Wednesday Day 32 4km Run (2.48 miles) 5k Plan 8km Run (4.97 miles) 10k Plan 85-90% of the Max Effort Baseline 6x-Av²/ci (Low Intensity) *Cross Exercise Training*	Wednesday Day 39 3km Run (1.86 miles) 5k Plan 6km Run (3.7 miles) 10k Plan At 70% of the Max Effort Baseline 6x-Av²/ci (Low Intensity) *Cross Exercise Training*
Thursday Day 33 3km Run (1.86 miles) 5k Plan 6km Run (3.7 miles) 10k Plan At 90% of max Effort Baseline 4x-Av²/ci (Low Intensity) *Cross Exercise Training*	Thursday Day 40 2km Run (1.2 miles) 5k Plan 4km Run (2.48 miles) 10k Plan At 75% of the Max Effort Baseline 4x-Av²/ci (Low Intensity) *Cross Exercise Training*
Friday Day 34 Run (Optional) Av²/ci (Optional)	Friday Day 41 Complete Rest (Optional)
Saturday Day 35 5km Run/Walk (3.1 miles) 5k Plan 10km Run/Walk (6.2 miles) 10k Plan 60-80% of the Max Effort Baseline Av²/ci *Cross Exercise Training Optional*	Saturday Day 42 Race Day: 5k or 10k Good Luck

TwQ 6 x10^3 Algorithm Time Key

See instructions below for calculating averages of:

One Mile Splits
One Kilometer Splits
Lap Splits
Rounds (or) Intervals

Refer to the chart with one-minute and one-hundredth time values from one minute to eight hours.
6 x10^3 = 6000 (1/100ths) = (One Minute TwQ Algorithm Key) mcw '13-22

The first step in the process is reducing the total exercise time to 1/100th. Refer to the following Example:

Example:

5-kilometer Race Day Finish time (21.48.79)
Step One: Remove the Decimals 21.48.79 to 21 48 79
Step Two: Calculate as: 21 x 6000 + 4879 = 130879 1/100ths

Now that the 5km (3.1 miles) time (21.48.79) has been reduced to a total of one-hundredths (130879), calculating for Average Kilometer, mile, track lap, and even miles per hour is a simple process using the time key value operation as follows:

Calculating For Average Kilometer:

130879 1/100ths ÷ by 5km = 26175.8 1/100ths
Refer to the time key value algorithm chart for finding a value less than 26175.8 (4 minutes = 24000 1/100ths)
26175.8 – 24000 (4) = 4.21.75 Average Kilometer Pace

Calculating for Average Mile:

130879 1/100ths ÷ by 3.1 = 42219 1/100ths
Refer to Time Key Value Algorithm Chart for finding a value less than 42219 (7 minutes = 42000 1/100ths)
42219 – 42000 (7) = 7.02.19 Average Mile Pace

"RUNNING IS THE POSITIVE PLACE I GO TO LEAVE THIS IMPRISONED REALITY!"
Heathen Warrior

Calculating Miles per hour (MPH):

Re: 5km Race Day Finish Time (21.48.79)
Convert 21.48.79 to total 1/100ths as on previous page
Step One: Remove the Decimals 21.48.79 to 21 48 79
Step Two: Calculate as: 21 x 6000 + 4879 = 130879 1/100ths

Miles Per Hour: 360000 1/100ths = 1 hour

Kilometers per hour:

Calculate as:

360000 ÷ 130879 = 2.7506
2.7506 multiplied by distance run:
2.7506 x 3.1 miles = 8.52 (mph)
2.7506 x 5km = 13.75 (kph)

Calculate For Average of a Ten round Cross Exercise Workout Performed in 60 minutes

60 minutes = 360000 1/100ths

Calculate as:

360000 ÷ by 10 Rounds = 36000 1/100ths
Refer to time Key Value Algorithm Chart for finding value less than (and/or) same as 36000 1/100ths

36000 1/100ths = 6 minutes = 6.00.00 Average Round

A versatile Conversion Algorithm with minutes and hundredths time Key chart that supports a value range:
From one minute = (6000 1/100ths)
To Eight hours = (2880000 1/100ths)

THIS 6 X 10^3 TwQ ALGORITHM MCW '13-'22 IS DEDICATED TO MY SONS TRISTIN HUNTER AND QUINTIN MATTHEW!

6 X 10^3 = 6,000 (1/100THS) =
(ONE MINUTE TWQ ALGORITHM KEY) MCW '13-22

Min/Hr	1/100ths	Min/Hr	1/100ths	Min/Hr	1/100ths	Min/Hr	1/100ths	Min/Hr	1/100ths
1	6000	49	294000	1:37.00	582000	2:25.00	870000	3:13.00	1158000
2	12000	50	300000	1:38.00	588000	2:26.00	876000	3:14.00	1164000
3	18000	51	306000	1:39.00	594000	2:27.00	882000	3:15.00	1170000
4	24000	52	312000	1:40.00	600000	2:28.00	888000	3:16.00	1176000
5	30000	53	318000	1:41.00	606000	2:29.00	894000	3:17.00	1182000
6	36000	54	324000	1:42.00	612000	2:30.00	900000	3:18.00	1188000
7	42000	55	330000	1:43.00	618000	2:31.00	906000	3:19.00	1194000
8	48000	56	336000	1:44.00	624000	2:32.00	912000	3:20.00	1200000
9	54000	57	342000	1:45.00	630000	2:33.00	918000	3:21.00	1206000
10	60000	58	348000	1:46.00	636000	2:34.00	924000	3:22.00	1212000
11	66000	59	354000	1:47.00	642000	2:35.00	930000	3:23.00	1218000
12	72000	1:00.00	360000	1:48.00	648000	2:36.00	936000	3:24.00	1224000
13	78000	1:01.00	366000	1:49.00	654000	2:37.00	942000	3:25.00	1230000
14	84000	1:02.00	372000	1:50.00	660000	2:38.00	948000	3:26.00	1236000
15	90000	1:03.00	378000	1:51.00	666000	2:39.00	954000	3:27.00	1242000
16	96000	1:04.00	384000	1:52.00	672000	2:40.00	960000	3:28.00	1248000
17	102000	1:05.00	390000	1:53.00	678000	2:41.00	966000	3:29.00	1254000
18	108000	1:06.00	396000	1:54.00	684000	2:42.00	972000	3:30.00	1260000
19	114000	1:07.00	402000	1:55.00	690000	2:43.00	978000	3:31.00	1266000
20	120000	1:08.00	408000	1:56.00	696000	2:44.00	984000	3:32.00	1272000
21	126000	1:09.00	414000	1:57.00	702000	2:45.00	990000	3:33.00	1278000
22	132000	1:10.00	420000	1:58.00	708000	2:46.00	996000	3:34.00	1284000
23	138000	1:11.00	426000	1:59.00	714000	2:47.00	1002000	3:35.00	1290000
24	144000	1:12.00	432000	2:00.00	720000	2:48.00	1008000	3:36.00	1296000
25	150000	1:13.00	438000	2:01.00	726000	2:49.00	1014000	3:37.00	1302000
26	156000	1:14.00	444000	2:02.00	732000	2:50.00	1020000	3:38.00	1308000
27	162000	1:15.00	450000	2:03.00	738000	2:51.00	1026000	3:39.00	1314000
28	168000	1:16.00	456000	2:04.00	744000	2:52.00	1032000	3:40.00	1320000
29	174000	1:17.00	462000	2:05.00	750000	2:53.00	1038000	3:41.00	1326000
30	180000	1:18.00	468000	2:06.00	756000	2:54.00	1044000	3:42.00	1332000
31	186000	1:19.00	474000	2:07.00	762000	2:55.00	1050000	3:43.00	1338000
32	192000	1:20.00	480000	2:08.00	768000	2:56.00	1056000	3:44.00	1344000
33	198000	1:21.00	486000	2:09.00	774000	2:57.00	1062000	3:45.00	1350000
34	204000	1:22.00	492000	2:10.00	780000	2:58.00	1068000	3:46.00	1356000
35	210000	1:23.00	498000	2:11.00	786000	2:59.00	1074000	3:47.00	1362000
36	216000	1:24.00	504000	2:12.00	792000	3:00.00	1080000	3:48.00	1368000
37	222000	1:25.00	510000	2:13.00	798000	3:01.00	1086000	3:49.00	1374000
38	228000	1:26.00	516000	2:14.00	804000	3:02.00	1092000	3:50.00	1380000
39	234000	1:27.00	522000	2:15.00	810000	3:03.00	1098000	3:51.00	1386000
40	240000	1:28.00	528000	2:16.00	816000	3:04.00	1104000	3:52.00	1392000
41	246000	1:29.00	534000	2:17.00	822000	3:05.00	1110000	3:53.00	1398000
42	252000	1:30.00	540000	2:18.00	828000	3:06.00	1116000	3:54.00	1404000
43	258000	1:31.00	546000	2:19.00	834000	3:07.00	1122000	3:55.00	1410000
44	264000	1:32.00	552000	2:20.00	840000	3:08.00	1128000	3:56.00	1416000
45	270000	1:33.00	558000	2:21.00	846000	3:09.00	1134000	3:57.00	1422000
46	276000	1:34.00	564000	2:22.00	852000	3:10.00	1140000	3:58.00	1428000
47	282000	1:35.00	570000	2:23.00	858000	3:11.00	1146000	3:59.00	1434000
48	288000	1:36.00	576000	2:24.00	864000	3:12.00	1152000	4:00.00	1440000

6×10^3 = 6,000 1/100THS = (ONE MINUTE TWO ALGORITHM KEY) MCW '13-22

Min/Hr	1/100ths	Min/Hr	1/100ths	Min/Hr	1/100ths	Min/Hr	1/100ths	Min/Hr	1/100ths
4:01.00	1446000	4:49.00	1734000	5:37.00	2022000	6:25.00	2310000	7:13.00	2598000
4:02.00	1452000	4:50.00	1740000	5:38.00	2028000	6:26.00	2316000	7:14.00	2604000
4:03.00	1458000	4:51.00	1746000	5:39.00	2034000	6:27.00	2322000	7:15.00	2610000
4:04.00	1464000	4:52.00	1752000	5:40.00	2040000	6:28.00	2328000	7:16.00	2616000
4:05.00	1470000	4:53.00	1758000	5:41.00	2046000	6:29.00	2334000	7:17.00	2622000
4:06.00	1476000	4:54.00	1764000	5:42.00	2052000	6:30.00	2340000	7:18.00	2628000
4:07.00	1482000	4:55.00	1770000	5:43.00	2058000	6:31.00	2346000	7:19.00	2634000
4:08.00	1488000	4:56.00	1776000	5:44.00	2064000	6:32.00	2352000	7:20.00	2640000
4:09.00	1494000	4:57.00	1782000	5:45.00	2070000	6:33.00	2358000	7:21.00	2646000
4:10.00	1500000	4:58.00	1788000	5:46.00	2076000	6:34.00	2364000	7:22.00	2652000
4:11.00	1506000	4:59.00	1794000	5:47.00	2082000	6:35.00	2370000	7:23.00	2658000
4:12.00	1512000	5:00.00	1800000	5:48.00	2088000	6:36.00	2376000	7:24.00	2664000
4:13.00	1518000	5:01.00	1806000	5:49.00	2094000	6:37.00	2382000	7:25.00	2670000
4:14.00	1524000	5:02.00	1812000	5:50.00	2100000	6:38.00	2388000	7:26.00	2676000
4:15.00	1530000	5:03.00	1818000	5:51.00	2106000	6:39.00	2394000	7:27.00	2682000
4:16.00	1536000	5:04.00	1824000	5:52.00	2112000	6:40.00	2400000	7:28.00	2688000
4:17.00	1542000	5:05.00	1830000	5:53.00	2118000	6:41.00	2406000	7:29.00	2694000
4:18.00	1548000	5:06.00	1836000	5:54.00	2124000	6:42.00	2412000	7:30.00	2700000
4:19.00	1554000	5:07.00	1842000	5:55.00	2130000	6:43.00	2418000	7:31.00	2706000
4:20.00	1560000	5:08.00	1848000	5:56.00	2136000	6:44.00	2424000	7:32.00	2712000
4:21.00	1566000	5:09.00	1854000	5:57.00	2142000	6:45.00	2430000	7:33.00	2718000
4:22.00	1572000	5:10.00	1860000	5:58.00	2148000	6:46.00	2436000	7:34.00	2724000
4:23.00	1578000	5:11.00	1866000	5:59.00	2154000	6:47.00	2442000	7:35.00	2730000
4:24.00	1584000	5:12.00	1872000	6:00.00	2160000	6:48.00	2448000	7:36.00	2736000
4:25.00	1590000	5:13.00	1878000	6:01.00	2166000	6:49.00	2454000	7:37.00	2742000
4:26.00	1596000	5:14.00	1884000	6:02.00	2172000	6:50.00	2460000	7:38.00	2748000
4:27.00	1602000	5:15.00	1890000	6:03.00	2178000	6:51.00	2466000	7:39.00	2754000
4:28.00	1608000	5:16.00	1896000	6:04.00	2184000	6:52.00	2472000	7:40.00	2760000
4:29.00	1614000	5:17.00	1902000	6:05.00	2190000	6:53.00	2478000	7:41.00	2766000
4:30.00	1620000	5:18.00	1908000	6:06.00	2196000	6:54.00	2484000	7:42.00	2772000
4:31.00	1626000	5:19.00	1914000	6:07.00	2202000	6:55.00	2490000	7:43.00	2778000
4:32.00	1632000	5:20.00	1920000	6:08.00	2208000	6:56.00	2496000	7:44.00	2784000
4:33.00	1638000	5:21.00	1926000	6:09.00	2214000	6:57.00	2502000	7:45.00	2790000
4:34.00	1644000	5:22.00	1932000	6:10.00	2220000	6:58.00	2508000	7:46.00	2796000
4:35.00	1650000	5:23.00	1938000	6:11.00	2226000	6:59.00	2514000	7:47.00	2802000
4:36.00	1656000	5:24.00	1944000	6:12.00	2232000	7:00.00	2520000	7:48.00	2808000
4:37.00	1662000	5:25.00	1950000	6:13.00	2238000	7:01.00	2526000	7:49.00	2814000
4:38.00	1668000	5:26.00	1956000	6:14.00	2244000	7:02.00	2532000	7:50.00	2820000
4:39.00	1674000	5:27.00	1962000	6:15.00	2250000	7:03.00	2538000	7:51.00	2826000
4:40.00	1680000	5:28.00	1968000	6:16.00	2256000	7:04.00	2544000	7:52.00	2832000
4:41.00	1686000	5:29.00	1974000	6:17.00	2262000	7:05.00	2550000	7:53.00	2838000
4:42.00	1692000	5:30.00	1980000	6:18.00	2268000	7:06.00	2556000	7:54.00	2844000
4:43.00	1698000	5:31.00	1986000	6:19.00	2274000	7:07.00	2562000	7:55.00	2850000
4:44.00	1704000	5:32.00	1992000	6:20.00	2280000	7:08.00	2568000	7:56.00	2856000
4:45.00	1710000	5:33.00	1998000	6:21.00	2286000	7:09.00	2574000	7:57.00	2862000
4:46.00	1716000	5:34.00	2004000	6:22.00	2292000	7:10.00	2580000	7:58.00	2868000
4:47.00	1722000	5:35.00	2010000	6:23.00	2298000	7:11.00	2586000	7:59.00	2874000
4:48.00	1728000	5:36.00	2016000	6:24.00	2304000	7:12.00	2592000	8:00.00	2880000

1Kilometer PR @ 100% Effort
Intensity/Training Percentage Zones

1k P.R.	95%	90%	85%	80%	75%	70%	65%	60%	1/100ths
2.30.00	2.37.89	2.46.66	2.56.47	3.07.50	3.20.00	3.34.28	3.50.76	4.10.00	15000
2.35.00	2.43.15	2.52.22	3.02.35	3.13.75	3.26.66	3.41.42	3.58.46	4.18.33	15500
2.40.00	2.48.42	2.57.77	3.08.23	3.20.00	3.33.33	3.48.57	4.06.15	4.26.66	16000
2.45.00	2.53.68	3.03.33	3.14.11	3.26.25	3.40.00	3.55.71	4.13.84	4.35.00	16500
2.50.00	2.58.94	3.08.88	3.20.00	3.32.50	3.46.66	4.02.85	4.21.53	4.43.33	17000
2.55.00	3.04.21	3.14.44	3.25.88	3.38.75	3.53.33	4.10.00	4.29.23	4.51.66	17500
3.00.00	3.09.47	3.20.00	3.31.76	3.45.00	4.00.00	4.17.14	4.36.92	5.00.00	18000
3.05.00	3.14.73	3.25.55	3.37.64	3.51.25	4.06.66	4.24.28	4.44.61	5.08.33	18500
3.10.00	3.20.00	3.31.11	3.43.52	3.57.50	4.13.33	4.31.42	4.52.30	5.16.66	19000
3.15.00	3.25.26	3.36.66	3.49.41	4.03.75	4.20.00	4.38.57	5.00.00	5.25.00	19500
3.20.00	3.30.52	3.42.22	3.55.29	4.10.00	4.26.66	4.45.71	5.07.69	5.33.33	20000
3.25.00	3.35.78	3.47.77	4.01.17	4.16.25	4.33.33	4.52.85	5.15.38	5.41.66	20500
3.30.00	3.41.05	3.53.33	4.07.05	4.22.50	4.40.00	5.00.00	5.23.07	5.50.00	21000
3.35.00	3.46.31	3.58.88	4.12.94	4.28.75	4.46.66	5.07.14	5.30.76	5.58.33	21500
3.40.00	3.51.57	4.04.44	4.18.82	4.35.00	4.53.33	5.14.28	5.38.46	6.06.66	22000
3.45.00	3.56.84	4.10.00	4.24.70	4.41.25	5.00.00	5.21.42	5.46.15	6.15.00	22500
3.50.00	4.02.10	4.15.55	4.30.58	4.47.50	5.06.66	5.28.57	5.53.84	6.23.33	23000
3.55.00	4.07.36	4.21.11	4.36.47	4.53.75	5.13.33	5.35.71	6.01.53	6.31.66	23500
4.00.00	4.12.63	4.26.66	4.42.35	5.00.00	5.20.00	5.42.85	6.09.23	6.40.00	24000
4.05.00	4.17.89	4.32.22	4.48.23	5.06.25	5.26.66	5.50.00	6.16.92	6.48.33	24500
4.10.00	4.23.15	4.37.77	4.54.11	5.12.50	5.33.33	5.57.14	6.24.61	6.56.66	25000
4.15.00	4.28.42	4.43.33	5.00.00	5.18.75	5.40.00	6.04.28	6.32.30	7.05.00	25500
4.20.00	4.33.68	4.48.88	5.05.88	5.25.00	5.46.66	6.11.42	6.40.00	7.13.33	26000
4.25.00	4.38.94	4.54.44	5.11.76	5.31.25	5.53.33	6.18.57	6.47.69	7.21.66	26500
4.30.00	4.44.21	5.00.00	5.17.64	5.37.50	6.00.00	6.25.71	6.55.38	7.30.00	27000
4.35.00	4.49.47	5.05.55	5.23.52	5.43.75	6.06.66	6.32.85	7.03.07	7.38.33	27500
4.40.00	4.54.73	5.11.11	5.29.41	5.50.00	6.13.33	6.40.00	7.10.76	7.46.66	28000
4.45.00	5.00.00	5.16.66	5.35.29	5.56.25	6.20.00	6.47.14	7.18.46	7.55.00	28500
4.50.00	5.05.26	5.22.22	5.41.17	6.02.50	6.26.66	6.54.28	7.26.15	8.03.33	29000
4.55.00	5.10.52	5.27.77	5.47.05	6.08.75	6.33.33	7.01.42	7.33.84	8.11.66	29500
5.00.00	5.15.78	5.33.33	5.52.94	6.15.00	6.40.00	7.08.57	7.41.53	8.20.00	30000
5.05.00	5.21.05	5.38.88	5.58.82	6.21.25	6.46.66	7.15.71	7.49.23	8.28.33	30500
5.10.00	5.26.31	5.44.44	6.04.70	6.27.50	6.53.33	7.22.85	7.56.92	8.36.66	31000
5.15.00	5.31.57	5.50.00	6.10.58	6.33.75	7.00.00	7.30.00	8.04.61	8.45.00	31500
5.20.00	5.36.84	5.55.55	6.16.47	6.40.00	7.06.66	7.37.14	8.12.30	8.53.33	32000
5.25.00	5.42.10	6.01.11	6.22.35	6.46.25	7.13.33	7.44.28	8.20.00	9.01.66	32500
5.30.00	5.47.36	6.06.66	6.28.23	6.52.50	7.20.00	7.51.42	8.27.69	9.10.00	33000
5.35.00	5.52.63	6.12.22	6.34.11	6.58.75	7.26.66	7.58.57	8.35.38	9.18.33	33500
5.40.00	5.57.89	6.17.77	6.40.00	7.05.00	7.33.33	8.05.71	8.43.07	9.26.66	34000
5.45.00	6.03.15	6.23.33	6.45.88	7.11.25	7.40.00	8.12.85	8.50.76	9.35.00	34500
5.50.00	6.08.42	6.28.88	6.51.76	7.17.50	7.46.66	8.20.00	8.58.46	9.43.33	35000
5.55.00	6.13.38	6.34.44	6.57.64	7.23.75	7.53.33	8.27.14	9.06.15	9.51.66	35500
6.00.00	6.18.94	6.40.00	7.03.52	7.30.00	8.00.00	8.34.28	9.13.84	10.00.00	36000

Goal Pace Key For Estimated Finish Times

1.609km	.6214 mi.	1.8642 mi.	3.107 mi.	4.9712 mi.	6.214 mi.	12.428 mi.	21.081km
1 Mile	1km	3km	5km	8km	10km	20km	13.1 mi. H.M.
4.25.53	2.45.00	8.15.00	13.45.00	22.00.00	27.30.00	55.00.00	57.58.44
4.33.57	2.50.00	8.30.00	14.09.98	22.39.97	28.19.96	56.39.92	59.43.76
4.41.62	2.55.00	8.44.99	14.34.99	23.19.99	29.09.98	58.19.97	1:01.29
4.49.66	3.00.00	8.59.98	14.59.97	23.59.95	29.59.94	59.59.89	1:03.14
4.57.71	3.05.00	9.14.99	15.24.98	24.39.97	30.49.97	1:01.40	1:05.00
5.05.76	3.10.00	9.30.00	15.49.99	25.19.99	31.40.00	1:03.20	1:06.45
5.13.80	3.15.00	9.44.98	16.14.97	25.59.96	32.29.95	1:05.00	1:08.30
5.21.85	3.20.00	10.00.00	16.39.98	26.39.98	33.19.97	1:06.39	1:10.16
5.29.90	3.25.00	10.15.00	17.05.00	27.20.00	34.10.00	1:08.19	1:12.01
5.37.94	3.30.00	10.29.98	17.29.98	27.59.96	35.00.00	1:10.00	1:13.47
5.45.99	3.35.00	10.44.99	17.54.99	28.39.98	35.49.98	1:11.40	1:15.32
5.54.04	3.40.00	11.00.00	18.20.00	29.20.00	36.40.00	1:13.20	1:17.17
6.02.08	3.45.00	11.14.99	18.44.98	29.59.97	37.29.96	1:15.00	1:19.03
6.10.13	3.50.00	11.29.99	19.09.99	30.40.00	38.19.98	1:16.39	1:20.48
6.18.17	3.55.00	11.44.98	19.34.97	31.19.95	39.09.94	1:18.19	1:22.34
6.26.22	4.00.00	12.00.00	19.59.98	31.59.97	40.00.00	1:20.00	1:24.19
6.34.27	4.05.00	12.14.99	20.24.99	32.40.00	40.50.00	1:21.40	1:26.04
6.42.31	4.10.00	12.29.98	20.49.97	33.19.96	41.39.95	1:23.20	1:27.50
6.50.36	4.15.00	12.44.99	21.14.98	33.59.98	42.29.97	1:24.59	1:29.35
6.58.41	4.20.00	13.00.00	21.40.00	34.40.00	43.20.00	1:26.40	1:31.21
7.06.45	4.25.00	13.14.98	22.04.98	35.19.96	44.09.96	1:28.19	1:33.06
7.14.50	4.30.00	13.29.99	22.30.00	35.59.98	44.59.98	1:30.00	1:34.51
7.22.55	4.35.00	13.45.00	22.55.00	36.40.00	45.50.00	1:31.29	1:36.37
7.30.59	4.40.00	13.59.98	23.19.98	37.19.97	46.39.96	1:33.20	1:38.22
7.38.64	4.45.00	14.15.00	23.45.00	37.59.99	47.29.98	1:35.00	1:40.08
7.46.68	4.50.00	14.29.98	24.09.97	38.39.96	48.19.95	1:36.39	1:41.53
7.54.73	4.55.00	14.44.99	24.34.98	39.19.97	49.09.97	1:38.19	1:43.38
8.02.78	5.00.00	15.00.00	25.00.00	39.59.99	49.59.99	1:40.00	1:45.24
8.10.82	5.05.00	15.14.98	25.24.97	40.39.96	50.49.95	1:41.39	1:47.09
8.18.87	5.10.00	15.29.99	25.50.00	41.19.98	51.39.97	1:43.20	1:48.55
8.26.92	5.15.00	15.45.00	26.15.00	42.00.00	52.30.00	1:45.00	1:50.40
8.34.96	5.20.00	16.00.00	26.39.98	42.40.00	53.20.00	1:46.40	1:52.25
8.43.01	5.25.00	16.14.99	27.04.99	43.20.00	54.10.00	1:48.20	1:54.11
8.51.06	5.30.00	16.30.00	27.30.00	44.00.00	55.00.00	1:50.00	1:55.56
8.59.10	5.35.00	16.45.00	27.54.98	44.39.97	55.49.96	1:51.40	1:57.42
9.07.15	5.40.00	17.00.00	28.20.00	45.19.99	56.39.99	1:53.20	1:59.27
9.15.19	5.45.00	17.14.98	28.44.97	46.00.00	57.29.95	1:55.00	2:01.12
9.23.24	5.50.00	17.29.99	29.10.00	46.39.98	58.19.97	1:56.39	2:02.58
9.31.29	5.55.00	17.45.00	29.35.00	47.20.00	59.10.00	1:58.19	2:04.43
9.39.33	6.00.00	17.59.98	29.59.97	47.59.96	59.59.95	2:00.00	2:06.29
9.47.38	6.05.00	18.14.99	30.24.99	48.39.98	1:00.50	2:01.39	2:08.14
9.55.43	6.10.00	18.30.00	30.50.00	49.20.00	1:01.40	2:03.20	2:10.13
10.03.47	6.15.00	18.44.98	31.14.98	49.59.97	1:02.29	2:05.00	2:11.45
10.11.52	6.20.00	18.59.99	31.40.00	50.39.98	1:03.19	2:06.39	2:13.30
10.19.56	6.25.00	19.14.98	32.04.97	51.19.95	1:04.10	2:08.19	2:15.16
10.27.61	6.30.00	19.29.99	32.29.98	51.59.97	1:04.59	2:10.00	2:17.01
10.35.66	6.35.00	19.44.99	32.55.00	52.40.00	1:05.49	2:11.40	2:18.47
10.43.70	6.40.00	19.59.98	33.19.97	53.19.96	1:06.40	2:13.19	2:20.32
10.51.75	6.45.00	20.15.00	33.44.98	54.00.00	1:07.29	2:15.00	2:22.17
10.59.80	6.50.00	20.30.00	34.10.00	54.39.99	1:08.20	2:16.40	2:24.03
11.07.84	6.55.00	20.44.98	34.34.97	55.19.96	1:09.09	2:18.19	2:25.48
11.15.89	7.00.00	20.59.99	34.59.99	55.59.98	1:09.59	2:19.59	2:27.34
11.23.94	7.05.00	21.15.00	35.25.00	56.40.00	1:10.50	2:21.40	2:29.19

AVERAGE LEVEL OF INTENSITY (A.L.O.I)
PERCENTAGE OF PHYSICAL OUTPUT (P.O.P.O)

H-RATE MAX

	114	120	126	132	138	144	150	156	162	168	174	180	186	192	198	204
204	56%	59%	62%	65%	68%	70.5%	73.5%	76%	79%	82%	85%	88%	91%	94%	97%	100%
198	57.5%	61%	64%	67%	70%	73%	76%	79%	82%	85%	88%	91%	94%	97%	100%	
192	59%	62.5%	66%	69%	72%	75%	78%	81%	84%	88%	91%	94%	97%	100%		
186	61%	64.5%	68%	71%	74%	77%	81%	84%	87%	90%	94.5%	97%	100%			
180	63%	67%	70%	73%	77%	80%	83%	87%	90%	93%	97%	100%				
174	65.5%	69%	72%	76%	79%	83%	86%	90%	93%	96.5%	100%					
168	68%	71%	75%	78.5%	72%	86%	89%	93%	96%	100%						
162	70%	74%	78%	81%	85%	89%	93%	96%	100%							
156	73%	77%	81%	85%	88%	92%	96%	100%								
150	76%	80%	84%	88%	92%	96%	100%									
144	79%	83%	87.5%	92%	96%	100%										
138	83%	87%	95%	96%	100%											
132	86%	91%	95%	100%												
126	90%	95%	100%													
120	95%	100%														
114	100%		→	103%	107%	110%	113%	117%	120%	123%	126%					
				Plus Death Range over Hr/Mx:					"for each range of bpm over max"							

PERCENTAGE OF PHYSICAL OUTPUT (P.O.P.O)

Base line training zone for Hr/Mx (220/180 bpm subtract age) Age/Hrate (time trial HrMx#)		
220 = anaerobic (vs) 180 = aerobic		
20=200/160	32=188/148	44=176/136
21=199/159	33=187/147	45175/135
22=198/158	34=186/146	46=174/134
23=197/157	35=185/145	47=173/133
24=196/156	36=184/144	48=172/132
25=195/155	37=183/143	49=171/131
26=194/154	38=182/142	50=170/130
27=193/153	39=181/141	51=169/129
28=192/152	40=180/140	52=168/128
29=191/151	41=179/139	53=167/127
30=190/150	42=178/138	54=166/126
31=189/149	43=177/137	55=165/125
Current 1km Hr/Mx: Date of test:		

bpm conversion key:	
"10 second pulse rate x 6 = bpm"	
10=60	23=138
11=66	24=144
12=72	25=150
13=78	26=156
14=84	27=162
15=90	28=168
16=96	29=174
17=102	30=180
18=108	31=186
19=114	32=192
20=120	33=198
21=126	34=204
22=132	25=210

*FOR CARDIO MAX * Hr/Mx *211 - (.64 x AGE) = Max bpm		
* ADVANCED ATHLETES *		
20 = 198.2	40 = 185.4	60 = 172.6
22 = 196.9	42 = 184.1	62 = 171.3
24 = 195.6	44 = 182.8	64 = 170
26 = 194.36	46 = 181.56	66 = 168.76
28 = 193.1	48 = 180.3	68 = 167.5
30 = 191.8	50 = 179	70 = 166.2
32 = 190.5	52 = 177.7	72 = 164.9
34 = 189.2	54 = 176.4	74 = 163.6
36 = 187.96	56 = 175.16	76 = 162.36
38 = 186.7	58 = 173.9	78 = 161.1

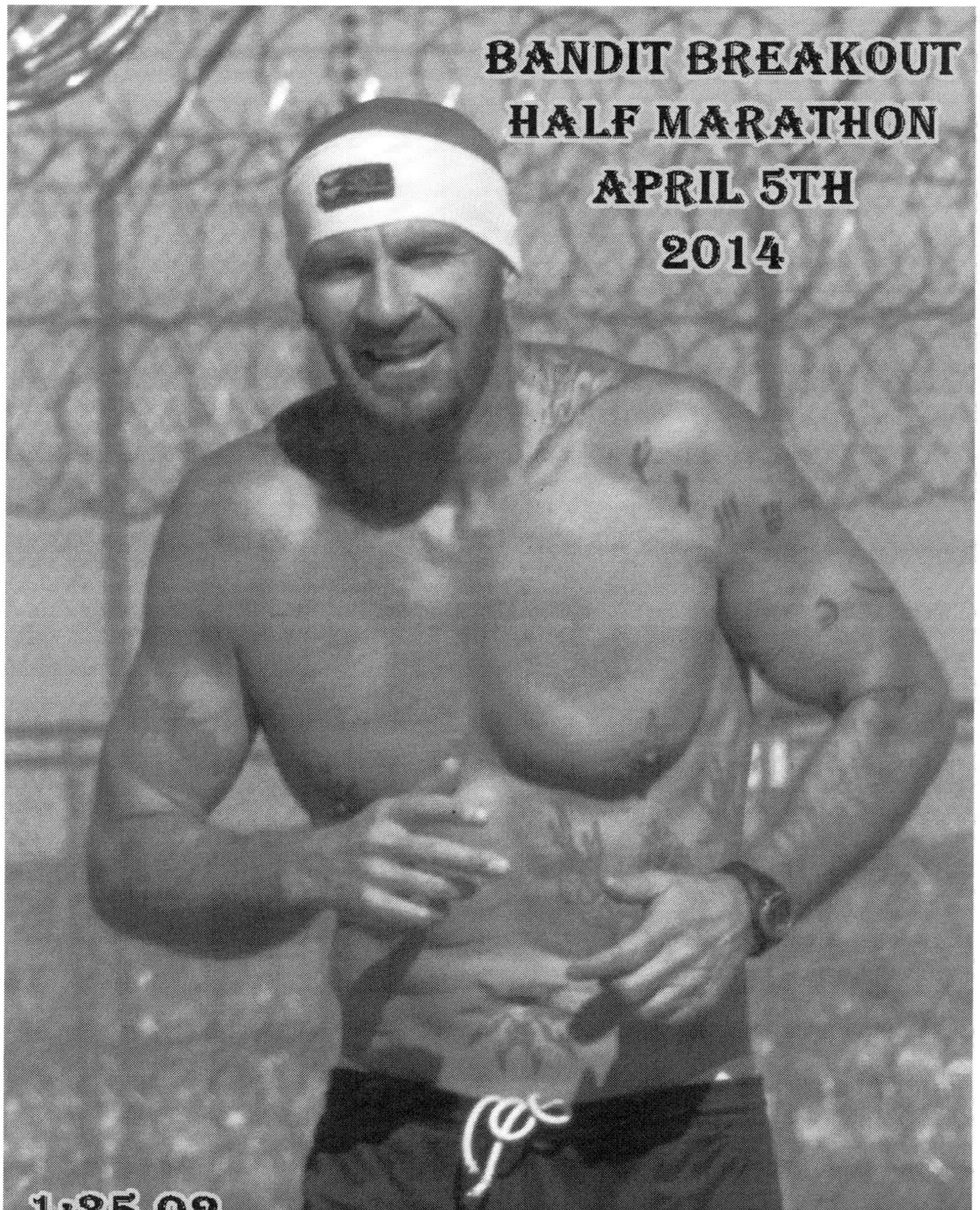
BANDIT BREAKOUT
HALF MARATHON
APRIL 5TH
2014
1:35.02

Section 6:

Heathen Chaos

&

Juggernäut Challenges

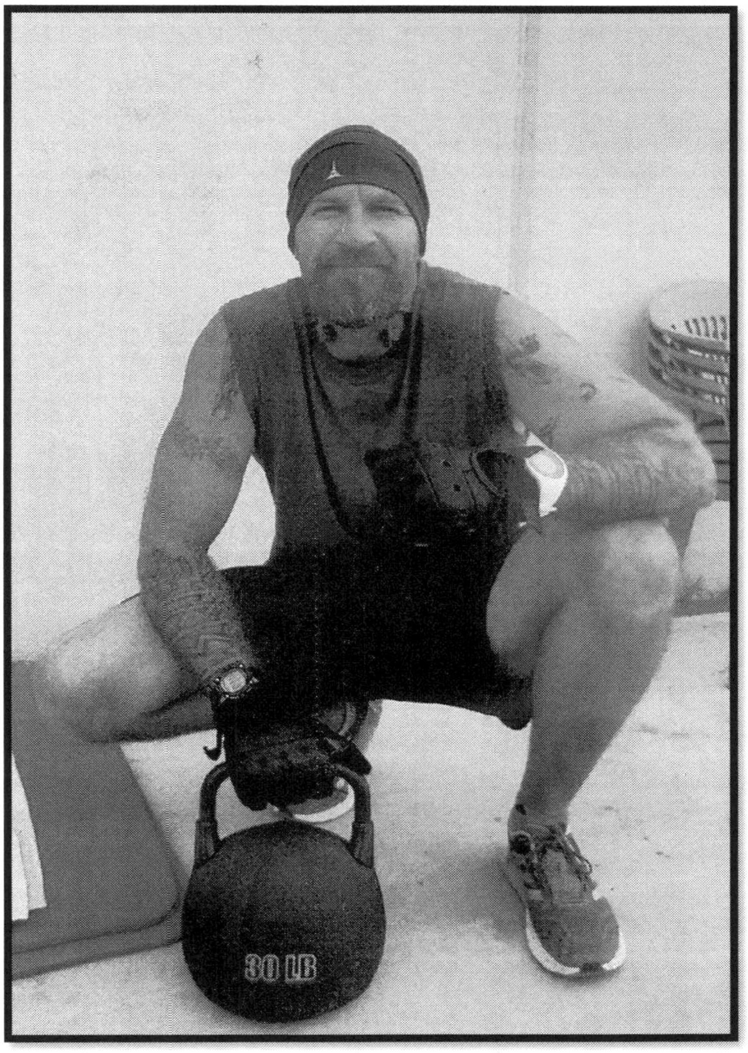

Heathen Chaos

Heathen Chaos consists of Running Intervals followed by a successive Cross Exercise Pyramid Set. There are two versions with five progression levels that increase both the running distance and the Rep count in the Cross Exercise Pyramid Set:

In version one, the level number dictates how many rounds of running 1-kilometer intervals and how many Reps to perform at each exercise in the Cross Exercise Pyramid Set.

In version two, the level number dictates the total run distance interval and how many Reps^2 (squared) to perform with each exercise in the Cross Exercise Pyramid Set.

The authors' Cross Exercise Pyramid Set consists of the following Five Exercises in a Pyramid order:

First:	**Muscle-ups**
Second:	**Toes to Bar**
Third:	**Kipping Handstand Push-up**
Fourth:	**DeadStop Burpee Jumping Jacks**
Fifth:	***Top of Pyramid requires Double Reps*** **90 Pound one-arm Gravity Squat-thrusters**
Sixth:	**DeadStop Burpee Jumping Jacks**
Seventh:	**Kipping Handstand Push-up**
Eighth:	**Toes to Bar**
Ninth:	**Muscle-up**

*Challenge yourself with the author's exercise order or tailor it to fit your abilities and work on weaknesses. The running Intervals are meant to Test Cardiovascular and Anaerobic Threshold Management before entering the Cross Exercise Pyramid Set. The Cross Exercise Pyramid Set also serves a sinister purpose during level progression. Cardio, anaerobic, and **Cross Exercise Repetition Threshold** management will be vital in completing each level without Resting Intervals, Tempo Management and Duration equals **Effort Intensity**. *

For beginners, scale down the author's five exercises that complement your **Fitness Level**. Blending the running discipline with Cross Exercise Repetition sets will prepare you for **Maximum Effort** finishes from four to sixty-minute workout durations. Evaluate your current Fitness Level before attempting these **Heathen Chaos Challenges**. What are your Strengths? What are your weaknesses? Embrace Both! We all began somewhere and at some level of training intensity. Be patient with the process involved in conditioning your body for Running Cross Exercise Interval Workouts.

The Following examples of Heathen Chaos are the authors' best benchmark finish times. Also included in the following examples is the workout date, time of day, weather information, Heart Rate, Effort Intensity Percentage, and Total Calorie Expense for the Reader to test his/her **Run Cross Exercise Efficiency Level.**

Heathen Chaos Version 1 Level 1

One Round of:

1. One Kilometer Run (.6214 mi) 2. One Rep Cross Exercise Pyramid Set	Workout Data June 17th, 2022, 9:30-10 AM Finish time @ 5.09.04 (PB) 180 BPM = 100% Effort Intensity Total Calorie Expense 77.9 Weather 95° Sunny w/35% humidity Total Run Distance .6214 mi (and) = 1km

Heathen Chaos Version 1 Level 2

Two Rounds of:

1. One Kilometer Run Interval (.6214 mi) 2. Two Rep Cross Exercise Pyramid Set	Workout Data June 17, 2022, 9-9:30 AM Finish Time @ 12.37.69 (PB) 168 BPM = 93% of HrMx Effort Intensity Total Calorie Expense 173.25 Weather 90° +/- Sunny w/35% Humidity Total Run Distance 2km (and) = 1.24 miles

Heathen Chaos Version 1 Level 3

Three Rounds of:

1. One Kilometer Run Interval (.6214 mi) 2. Three Rep Cross Exercise Pyramid Set	Workout Data April 12, 2022, 9-10 AM Finish Time @ 24.20.27 (PB) 168 BPM = 93% of HrMx Effort Intensity Total Calorie Expense 337.2 Weather 65°- 70° Sunny w/NW Wind @ 25 mph Total Run Distance 3km (and) = 1.86 Miles

Complete Instructional Example
Heathen Chaos Version 1 Level 4

Four Rounds of:

1.	One kilometer Run Interval (.6214 mi)	Workout Data April 1, 2022, 8-9 AM Finish time @ 39.49.59 (PB) 169 BPM = 94% of HrMx Effort Intensity Total Calorie Expense 558.8 Weather 60°- 65° Sunny and Nice! Total run Distance 4km (and) = 2.48 Miles
2.	Four Rep Cross Exercise Pyramid Set	
1.	One Kilometer Run Interval (.6214 mi)	
2.	Four Rep Cross Exercise Pyramid Set	
1.	One kilometer Run Interval (.6214 mi)	
2.	Four Rep Cross Exercise Pyramid Set	
1.	One kilometer Run Interval (.6214 mi)	
2.	Four Rep Cross Exercise Pyramid Set	

Authors Notes:

1km Run Time	4.07.39
4x Rep C.E.P.S.	5.38.29
Round 1 Total:	9.45.68
1km Run Time	4.19.62
4x Rep C.E.P.S.	5.25.17
Round 2 Total:	9.44.79
1km Run Time	4.20.09
4x Rep C.E.P.S.	5.39.68
Round 3 Total:	9.59.77
1km Run Time	4.24.54
4x Rep C.E.P.S.	5.54.81
Round 4 Total:	10.19.35

Heathen Chaos Version 1 Level 5

Five Rounds of:

1.	One kilometer Run Interval (.6214 mi)	Workout Data March 14, 2022, 8-9 AM Finish time @ 59.47.61 (PB) 169 BPM = 94% of HrMx Effort Intensity Total Calorie Expense 839.6 Weather 55°- 60° Cool and Sunny Total Run Distance 5km = 3.1 Miles
2.	Five Rep Cross Exercise Pyramid Set	

Heathen Chaos Version 2 Level 1

Total Run and Total Rep² Squared Intervals:

1. One-kilometer total Run Interval (1km=.6214 mi) 2. Total One Rep² Cross Exercise Pyramid Set	Workout Data June 17, 2022, 9:30-10 AM Finish time @ 5.09.04 (PB) 180 BPM = 100% of HrMx Effort Intensity Total Calorie Expense 77.9 Weather 95° Sunny w/35% Humidity Total Run Distance 1km = .6214 Mile

Heathen Chaos Version 2 Level 2

Total Run and Total Rep² Squared Exercise Intervals:

1. Two-kilometer total Run Interval (2km= 1.24 mi) 2. Total Two Rep² Squared (4) Cross Exercise Pyramid Set	Workout Data May 5, 2022, 8-9 AM Finish Time @ 12.31.38 (PB) 168 BPM = 93% of HrMx Effort Intensity Total Calorie Expense 173.25 Weather 75° Sunny Total Run Distance 2km = 1.24 Miles

Heathen Chaos Version 2 Level 3

Total Run and Total Rep² Squared Exercise Intervals:

1. Three-kilometer total Run Interval (3km = 1.86 mi)	Workout Data May 8, 2022, 9-10 AM Finish time @ 26.20.95 (PB) 174 BPM = 96% of HrMx Effort Intensity Total Calorie Expense 379.4 Weather 80° Sunny Total run Distance 3km = 1.86 Miles

Heathen Chaos Version 2 Level 4

Total Run and Total Rep² Squared Exercise Intervals:

1.	Four-kilometer Total Run Interval (4km = 2.48 miles)	Author's Notes: 1. 4km Run time: 17.20.65 180 BPM = 100% HrMx
2.	Total Four Rep² (16) Cross Exercise Pyramid Set	2. 4² = 16x Total Rep Cross Exercise Pyramid Set Time: 29.39.78 168 BPM = 93% of HrMx

4² Squared Total Rep Pyramid Set Example:

1st	16x Reps	Muscle-ups	
2nd	16x Reps	Toes to Bar	
3rd	16x Reps	Kipping Handstand Push-ups	Workout Data
4th	16x Reps	DeadStop Burpee Jumping Jacks	May 7, 2022, 8-9 AM Finish Time @ 47.00.43 (PB)
Note: Double Reps at the top of Pyramid			174 BPM = 96% of HrMx Effort Intensity
5th	32x Reps	90lb one-arm Gravity Squat-thrusters	Total Calorie Expense 676.8 Weather 75°- 80° Sunny
6th	16x Reps	DeadStop Burpee Jumping Jacks	Total Run Distance 4km = 2.48 Miles
7th	16x Reps	Kipping Handstand Push-ups	
8th	16x Reps	Toes to Bar	
9th	16x Reps	Muscle-ups	

Heathen Chaos Version 2 Level 5

Total Run and Total Rep² Squared Exercise Interval:

1.	5km Total Run Interval (5km = 3.1 Miles) Total 5 Rep² Squared (25) Cross Exercise Pyramid Set	Workout Data July 16, 2022, 8-9 AM Finish Time @ 1:01.58 (PB) 165.6 BPM = 92% of HrMx Effort Intensity Total Calorie Expense 848.2 Weather 100° +/- Sunny w/45% Humidity Total run Distance 5km = 3.1 Miles

Versions One and Two have the same Total Distance in the Running Interval and Total Rep volume in The Cross Exercise Pyramid Set.
However similar the two versions and levels are, executing each is quite different in that both offer unique challenges dependent upon the Athletes Cross Exercise Efficiency Fitness Level.

Juggernäut Challenge
aka JugNäut

Please Note: Apply the With Run (WR-10) equation to your Effort Intensity Level/Zones and Calorie Expense calculations. Use this Challenge workout for monitoring current Cross Exercise Efficiency (CEE)Levels. Whether Advanced, Intermediate, or Beginner, it works excellent for logging weekly mileage as you progress in the Running and the Cross Exercise Rep Ascension Circuit Phases. **IT IS SIMPLE AND SIMPLY CHALLENGING!**

Tempo Equals Intensity

On the one hand, taking your time running through Phase I and Repping out the Cross Exercise Rep ascension Phase will still have great training benefits during Low-Intensity.

OR

Blasting through both phases like a mad woman/mad man, whoever you are, seeking a new personal best time, Max Effort Intensity (IE), Max Heart Rate, or burning full Expense of Calories...**This challenge is for you!**

Here's the objective in tracking the JugNäut Challenge. See the authors' Apex 8km JugNäut challenge Data for an instruction example.

***Note: The distance in kilometers you choose for challenges also dictates the number of Reps you perform for the first exercise in Phase II. ***

If you create your exercise line-up in Phase II to complement your abilities, it is essential to remember that Phase I should be your run, followed by Phase II Cross Exercise Rep Ascension Circuit.

Phase I (running) and Phase II (cross exercise reps) in this challenge is intended to tax the relationship between all three primary THRESHOLDS:

Cardiovascular (HrMx)

Pulmonary/Anaerobic (Vo2)

Muscular Endurance (m.e.t.)

As you progress, by adding distance in Phase I and faster cross-exercise rep tempo in Phase II, you will experience physical and mental confidence as you learn how to manage individual intensity thresholds. Enjoy the SUCK!

***Take Recovery only as needed and remember to log your Heart Rate (BPM) Beats Per Minute immediately upon finishing Phase I and Phase II. This information is valuable for Tracking/Documenting Effort Intensity Level Zones and Calorie Expenses. ***

Author's Actual Apex 8km JugNäut Challenge

Note: Apex is the highest level, and my Personal Apex personal Best Performing the JugNäut Challenge is 8 kilometers

Phase I:		8-kilometer Run
Phase II:		Cross Exercise Rep Ascend Circuit
*1.	8x Reps	Muscle-ups
2.	5x Reps	Kipping Handstand Push-ups
3.	10x Reps	DeadStop Burpee Jumping Jacks
4.	15x Reps	Strict Pull-ups
5.	20x Reps	Squat Thrusters
6.	25x Reps	Toes to Bars
7.	30x Reps	DeadStop Burpee Jumping Jacks
8.	35x Reps	Back Extensions
9.	40x Reps	Deep Body Squats
10.	5x Reps	Kipping Handstand Push-ups
*11.	8x Reps	Muscle-ups

Workout Data
February 8, 2022, 8-9 AM
Phase I Time @ 34.03.81
Phase II Time @ 21.18.87
Total Time: 55.22.68
168 BPM HrMx 93%
Effort Intensity Max Level/Zone 2
Calorie Expense @ 767.5
Weather 45°-50° Sunny
Run Distance 8km = 4.97 Miles

The data below is the author's Personal Best Workout Challenge Stats from the 1km JugNäut to the 8km JugNäut Apex. The information shows the readers how Tempo, Temperature, Humidity, and Challenge Duration affect Effort Intensity and Calorie Expenses.

*Cross Exercise Rep Ascension Circuit (C.E.R.A.C.) *

5km JugNäut Challenge Data
Phase I:
5km Run Time 20.48.73
Phase II:
C.E.R.A.C. Time 21.42.28
Total Finish Time
@ 42.49.53

Workout Data:
January 8, 2022, 8-9 AM
168 BPM = 93% of HrMx
Effort Intensity @ Max Zone 2
Calorie Expense @ 593.56
Weather 50°- 55° Sunny

7km JugNäut Challenge Data
Phase I:
7km Run Time 30.19.80
Phase II:
C.E.R.A.C. Time 24.20.62
Total Finish Time @ 54.41.42

Workout Data:
March 1, 2022, 9-10 AM
165 BPM = 92% of HrMx
Effort Intensity @ Max Zone 2
Calorie Expense @ 748.15
Weather 55°- 65° Sunny

6km JugNäut Challenge Data

Phase I:	Workout Data:
6km Run Time 24.41.86	March 26, 2022, 8-9 AM
Phase II:	167 BPM = 93% of HrMx
C.E.R.A.C. Time 21.51.32	Effort Intensity @ Max Zone 2
Total Finish Time @ 47.33.18	Calorie Expense @ 659.1
	Weather 65°- 75° Sunny

The author performed the final four JugNäut Challenges on four consecutive days to evaluate Outdoor Temperature and Humidity Effects on the Body even when the Duration is Relatively Short.

4km JugNäut Challenge Data

Phase I:	Workout Data:
4km Run Time 17.16.01	June 20, 2022, 8-9 AM
Phase II:	180 BPM = Max 100%
C.E.R.A.C. Time 22.15.73	Effort Intensity @ Max Zone 1
	Calorie Expense @ 597.67
Total Finish Time @ 39.31.74	Weather 91° w/41% Humidity

3km JugNäut Challenge Data

Phase I:	Workout Data:
3km Run Time 12.50.26	June 21, 2022, 9-10 AM
Phase II:	169 BPM = 94% of HrMx
C.E.R.A.C. Time 21.36.09	Effort Intensity @ Max Zone 2
	Calorie Expense @ 483.5
Total Finish Time @ 34.26:35	Weather 95.5° w/41% Humidity

Authors Actual 2km JugNäut Challenge

Phase I:	2 Kilometer Run	Workout Data
Phase II:	C.E.R.A.C.	June 22, 2022, 8-9 AM
*1. 2x Reps	Muscle-ups	Phase I Time 8.21.18
2. 5x Reps	Kipping Handstand Push-ups	Phase II Time 20.03.41
		Total Time 28.24.59
3. 10x Reps	DeadStop Burpee Jumping Jacks	169 BPM = 94% of HrMx
		Effort Intensity Max Zone 2
4. 15x Reps	Strict Pull-ups	Calorie Expense 398.9
5. 20x Reps	Squat Thrusters	Weather 95° w/50% Humidity
6. 25x Reps	Toes to Bar	Run Distance 2km = 1.24 Miles
7. 30x Reps	DeadStop Burpee Jumping Jacks	*Asterisk Represents the 2km Run that dictates the number of Reps in Exercise 1. 2x Reps (Muscle-ups and Exercise 11. 2x Reps (Muscle-ups).
8. 35x Reps	Back Extensions	
9. 40x Reps	Deep Body Squats	
10. 5x Reps	Kipping Handstand Push-ups	
*11. 2x Reps	Muscle-ups	

1km JugNäut Challenge Data

Phase I:	Workout Data
1km Run Time 3.55.81	June 23, 2022, 9-10 AM
Phase II:	168 BPM = 93% of HrMx
C.E.R.A.C. Time 19.28.25	Effort Intensity Max Zone 2
Total Finish Time @ 23.24.06	Calorie Expense @ 324.3
	Weather 100° w/35% Humidity

"I Do Not Follow Man! I Lead By Example With The Science and Evolution of Mental, Physical and Mechanical Health."

Heathen Warrior

Section Z:

Av^2/ci "Anaerobic Vo2 Cardio Intervals"

&

Av^2/ci "24-Day Training Plan"

Av^2/ci "Anaerobic Vo2 Cardio Intervals"

A quick history of how "Anaerobic Vo2 Cardio Intervals" became my primary Exercise routine in 2013.

The Av^2/ci Exercise routine began as "Hybrid Vo2 Intervals" (HvI's) 2.40.00/1.20.00 Exercise to recovery 2/1 ratio. **Hence: (HvI's) mcw est. '13.**

Ana/Vo2 Cardio Intervals (Av^2/ci) are the upgrade re-created in 2014 when I applied the routine specifically focused on competition training for the first time. This 2/1 ratio Exercise to recovery (3.00.00/1.30.00) became the recipe for success.

"Anaerobic Threshold Combined with Maximal Oxygen uptake (Vo2), is a Key Indicator for Cardiovascular Conditioning. The relationship is like upgrading a High-Performance Vehicle with a more Efficient and Powerful Engine."

The Av^2/ci "24-Day see the evolution of fitness cycle" and 5km running plan also came about as a result of success in 2015. The game changer was experiencing higher Rep volume in all Exercises and more efficient run intervals with lower post Exercise Heart Rate. Seeing my Evolution of Conditioning Performance and overall cross Exercise fitness sparked an interest in Exercise Physiology.

Note:
During my 24-Day Av^2/ci Training plan, as an individual progresses in fitness conditioning throughout the 24-days, that progress can be measured by a higher three-minute interval Rep volume. Av^2/ci works like this: An Individual has three minutes to run as far as possible in that strict amount of time. During that 24-day plan, most people can only run so far in three minutes. The fitter that person becomes and the faster they become, naturally, they cover more distance creating more efficient run intervals.

I began studying the subject while simultaneously applying the Sciences' as I progressed through the information. The Science of Fitness made so much sense. I started documenting every detail when performing the Av^2/ci routines…Post-interval Heart Rate (Beats Per Minute) Rep Volume, Duration of Workout, Weather Conditions (IE) Temperature, and Humidity Effects on Performance.

Performing any Exercise for three minutes, in a designated number of intervals in a sequence, will make learning to be mechanically efficient much more expedient.

"Applying the Av^2/ci. Routine to any Exercise is a straightforward process. Shift to the desired Exercises for specific training and competitive needs and perform the routine 24 days prior to a goal or event."

I am writing this Manual in an Arizona Private Contract Prison serving the Idaho Department of Correction Time mid-Year 2022. There are no fitness competitions here at this facility to test conditioning. Therefore, the Av^2/ci routine has been my primary workout four to seven times per week, ranging from four to thirteen intervals with all Exercise from Muscle-ups and Jumping Jacks to Running.

Credit due to the Av²/ci training routine, I have been able to maintain the following Personal Benchmarks here at this Arizona Facility:

- **19.52.89 5-Kilometer Run Time**
- **42.23.24 10-Kilometer Run Time**
- **See: "Heathen Chaos and Juggernäut Challenge Benchmark Personal best" Data in this Manual Section 6**
- **Muscle-ups Max Reps (No Partition) 18x (PB/Arizona) S.F.G.**
- **Muscle-ups Max Reps (No Partition) 11x (PB/Arizona N.S.R.G.**
- **Muscle-ups/Toes to Bar combination 15x R each without leaving the bar**
- **At 5:30 AM this morning on July 27th, 2022, I completed a 5km Run in 21.03.93. *Weather info: 85° F w/62% Humidity***
- **I am a 49-Year-old Blue Eyed Heathen Warrior with Peckerwood Chrome in my Beard. Age is only a number; the Chrome has been earned with Pride…16 1/2 years in the books easy, and the 8 ½ years to Freedom debt paid will also come to pass. What a Great Fucking Journey!**

An extensive amount of Science and Exercise Physiology never seems to find its way into the mainstream. Unfortunately, I feel like I am part of that same problem unless I do my best to change that by sharing this excellent training tool with the world and all the data collected over the last nine years utilizing all the potential this Av²/ci Exercise routine possesses.

Simple Breakdown of How to Apply this Av²/ci Routine:
Use the included Av²/ci Workout Sheets in this Manual's Calendar Log for Tracking Fitness/ Conditioning Progress.

Note:
Before beginning this Av²/ci training routine, it is necessary to acquire a Watch Or any device with a chronograph. An accurate fitness watch with a timer and Heart Rate monitor is ideal. The timer is needed to easily monitor the (3.00.00) Exercise Interval and the (1.30.00) Recovery Interval. This is for strict data tracking of Heart Rate and Exercise Max volume log entries.
Choose one to Twelve Exercises that will be performed in this sequence of intervals.

***SEE 4x-Av²/ci Example**

Example: Four Interval Sequence

Jumping Jacks	**3.00.00 (Max Reps)**	**1.30.00 Recovery**	**Log Data**
Run	**3.00.00 (Max Time)**	**1.30.00 Recovery**	**Log Data**
Rowing	**3.00.00 (Max Strokes)**	**1.30.00 Recovery**	**Log Data**
Cycle	**3.00.00 (Max Time)**	**Total Time Finish @ 16.30.00**	

First: Immediately upon completing the three-minute Exercise interval, log your Heart Rate, either from an accurate Heart Rate monitor or a self-check pulse for a strict 10 seconds at the subclavian artery located at the point inside where the collarbone meets the neck. *10 second pulse rate multiplied by 6 = (BPM) Beats Per Minute* Log Exercise Data as well for tracking.

Second: Perform a strict 1.30.00 Recovery Interval preparing for the next Exercise.

Efficient Cross Exercise Rep Volume Management during the three-minute interval followed by the strict 1.30.00 Recovery Interval will keep post-Exercise Heart Rate data more accurate when calculating Effort Intensity and Calorie Expense for Post Total Workout.

To find the Average Level Of Intensity (A.L.O.I.) when completing a routine
Baseline Heart Rate Max formulas:
220 subtract Age =
Note:
For Advanced Cardio/ Vo2 athletes **211 subtract .64 multiplied by Age Equals**

Add all Interval Heart Rate in (BPM) entries together and divide by the total number of Intervals Performed with (BPM) entries. This equates to an Average Heart Rate.
Now Divide your Average Heart Rate by your Max Heart Rate. This percentage is for calculating Effort Intensity. With/ KCal Value and Calorie Expense.
*Refer to Section 4 of this Manual, "Calculating Effort Intensity and Calorie Expenses."
* *Calorie Expense Variance*

Cross Exercises "With Run (WR-10)" Intervals
VERSUS
Cross Exercise "No Run (NR-10.8)" Intervals

Miscellaneous information below showing the Variance of Calorie Expenses when Performing ANA Vo2/Cardio Intervals:

- **With Run (WR-10)**
- **No Run (NR-10.8)**

Both Examples Represent Identical Stats in Gender, Age, Bodyweight, and Age-Related heart Rate max as Follows:

Woman, Age 35, Bodyweight 145 Pounds, Heart Rate max @ 185 BPM
8x-Av²/ci Routine Performed (Both Examples), Total Time to Complete 34.30.00 (34.5 Minutes), Average Level of Intensity (ALOI) @ 168 BPM – 90%, Effort Intensity 90% Level 2 High Zone 1.

1st 8x-Av²/ci With Run (WR-10)

Effort Intensity 90% KCal Value .74
Calculate .74 x Bodyweight (145) ÷ (WR-10) – 10.73 KCal Per Minute
10.73 x Duration of Workout (34.5) = 370.18 Total Calorie Expense

2nd 8x-Av²/ci No Run (NR-10.8)

Effort Intensity 90% KCal Value .74
Calculate .74 x Bodyweight (145) ÷ (NR-10.8) = 9.93 KCal Per minute
9.93 x Duration of Workout (34.5) = 342.76 Total Calorie Expense

A 27.42 Calorie Expense Variance

***Tempo Equals Intensity**
&
Duration of Interval (s)*

Choose the Level of Intensity for any Exercise Discipline:

- Running Laps for Max Time and Distance at Low to Maximum Effort
- Cross Exercise Strength Training Rep threshold for Max Time at Low to Maximum Effort (All Muscle Groups)
- Cycling for Distance or max Time at Low to Maximum Effort
- Rowing Machine Stroke Reps for Distance or max Time Rep Threshold at Low to Maximum Effort
- Swimming Laps for Distance or Max Time at Low to Maximum Effort

See the Example Below:

Tempo Equals Intensity and Duration of Interval (s)
RE: 8x-Av²/ci Routine *Av²/ci Interval Time Totals*

	Exercise Interval 3.00.00
1st	Spartan Burpee's: 15x Reps Total 144 BPM
	Recovery Interval 1.30.00
	Exercise Interval 3.00.00
2nd	Run: .25 miles Total 132 BPM
	Recovery Interval 1.30.00
	Exercise Interval 3.00.00
3rd	Rowing Machine: 90 Stroke Reps Total 144 BPM
	Recovery Interval 1.30.00
	Exercise Interval 3.00.00
4th	Stationary (Cycle): Low Tempo Total 132 BPM
	Recovery Interval 1.30.00
	Exercise Interval 3.00.00
5th	Spartan Burpee's: 40x Reps Total 174 BPM
	Recovery Interval 1.30.00
	Exercise Interval 3.00.00
6th	Run: .5 Miles Total 180 BPM
	Recovery Interval 1.30.00
	Exercise Interval 3.00.00
7th	Rowing Machine: 130 Stroke Reps Total 174 BPM
	Recovery Interval 1.30.00
8th	Exercise Interval 3.00.00
	Stationary (Cycle): Max Tempo total 174 BPM
Complete Total Time 34.30.00	

Choose the Number of Av²/ci 3.00.00 Exercise Intervals you wish to Perform, meeting individual time constraints around daily Activities. Complete with 1.30.00 Recovery Interval Totals in Strict Time Sequence:

1	3.00.00	Interval	(Exercise)	=	3.00.00
	1.30.00	Interval	(Recovery)	=	4.30.00
2	3.00.00	Interval	(Exercise)	=	7.30.00
	1.30.00	Interval	(Recovery)	=	9.00.00
3	3.00.00	Interval	(Exercise)	=	12.00.00
	1.30.00	Interval	(Recovery)	=	13.30.00
4	3.00.00	Interval	(Exercise)	=	16.30.00
	1.30.00	Interval	(Recovery)	=	18.00.00
5	3.00.00	Interval	(Exercise)	=	21.00.00
	1.30.00	Interval	(Recovery)	=	22.30.00
6	3.00.00	Interval	(Exercise)	=	25.30.00
	1.30.00	Interval	(Recovery)	=	27.00.00
7	3.00.00	Interval	(Exercise)	=	30.00.00
	1.30.00	Interval	(Recovery)	=	31.30.00
8	3.00.00	Interval	(Exercise)	=	34.30.00
	1.30.00	Interval	(Recovery)	=	36.00.00

9	3.00.00	Interval	(Exercise)	=	39.00.00
	1.30.00	Interval	(Recovery)	=	40.30.00
10	3.00.00	Interval	(Exercise)	=	43.30.00
	1.30.00	Interval	(Recovery)	=	45.00.00
11	3.00.00	Interval	(Exercise)	=	48.00.00
	1.30.00	Interval	(Recovery)	=	49.30.00
12	3.00.00	Interval	(Exercise)	=	52.30.00
	1.30.00	Interval	(Recovery)	=	54.00.00
13	3.00.00	Interval	(Exercise)	=	57.00.00
	1.30.00	Interval	(Recovery)	=	58.30.00
14	3.00.00	Interval	(Exercise)	=	1:01.30
	1.30.00	Interval	(Recovery)	=	1:03.00
15	3.00.00	Interval	(Exercise)	=	1:06.00

Note: There is no Recovery Interval when Completing the Last Exercise Interval in the Av²/ci Routine

Av²/ci 24-Day Training Plan

See the Evolution of Fitness…

Precautionary Note

It is imperative that you know your Physical Aptitude before Committing to this Training Plan.

Please Ask these Questions:

First: Do I know my max heart Rate (MxHr)?

220 – Age Equals (MxHr)

180 – Age Equals .76% of (MxHr)

Second: Do I know my physical Limitations?

Address and Assess any mechanical or medical issues before Beginning and Choose Exercises that Compliment your Individual Abilities.

Third: Am I familiar with the Exercises Chosen for 24 Days?

If the Exercises chosen are unfamiliar, be patient in allowing time for the Body to Adapt.

Practice any unfamiliar Exercises outside this Training Plan before the Training Plan Begins.

Prepare your Body!

Instructions:

This Training Plan is Unique in that it Incorporates Maximum, High, and Low Effort Intensity Levels Throughout each Three-Day Training Cycle.

Refer to the Chart in Section 4 of this Manual for Precise Effort Intensity Levels and Zones

Tracking daily data is extremely important in showing progress. Log Exercise Reps, Run Distance, and Post Exercise Interval Heart Rates, as this information will repeatedly change throughout the Duration of the training plan due to the body adapting to the daily Exercises.
Rep Count and Distance (Speed) Running benchmarks will increase, and Post Exercise Interval Heart Rates will decrease as higher Fitness Levels are Achieved.
Hence…. "Seeing the Evolution of Fitness."
Begin by choosing Eight Miscellaneous Exercises to Perform Every day for 24-Days.

Use the Example Below as a Reference:

Example:
8x-Av²/ci Exercise Order
Beginning order of the Training Cycle Begins at Max Intensity effort in all Eight Exercise Intervals to Establish a Baseline of Day #1 Benchmarks
As many Reps/Strokes as Possible

Max Distance Run 200 to 1200 Meters

1	**Jumping jacks**	5	**Sit-ups**
2	**Rowing Machine**	6	**Run**
3	**Push-ups**	7	**Rowing machine**
4	**Run**	8	**Burpee's**

Exercise Order Rotation Instructions:
Rotate the First Exercise in the Order (Jumping Jacks) to the Bottom of the Order in the Eighth Position. Repeat this at every Rotation of Order throughout the 24 days.

See First Rotation of Order Example

1	**Rowing Machine**	5	**Run**
2	**Push-ups**	6	**Rowing Machine**
3	**Run**	7	**Burpee's**
4	**Sit-ups**	8	**Jumping jacks**

There are Three Days per Cycle, each with Specific Training goals via a Full Range of Effort Intensities:

Day One of Three:

This is a Maximum Effort Intensity Workout to Establish Baseline Benchmark Numbers for each Interval of Exercises. **(Example)** Rowing Machine Max Effort Stroke Reps at (130 Stroke Reps) 100%.

Day Two of Three:

This is a Low Effort Intensity Active Recovery Workout. Perform the same Exercise order at 66% to 70% of the Current Rotation Baseline of Max Effort benchmarks (**Example)** Burpee Max Rep Effort at (45 Reps) 45 x 66% Equals 30 Burpee's.

Day Three of Three:

This is a High Effort Intensity Active Workout Engineered to Prepare the Body for Maximum Effort in the Successive Rotation. Perform the same order at 76% to 80% of the Current rotation Baseline of Max Effort Benchmarks. **(Example)** Run Max Distance Effort at (800 Meters) 800 x 80% Equals 640 Meters.

Simple Calculations for Percentage of Exercise Reps and Run Distance Goals:

Example:	**Jumping Jacks Max Rep Benchmark number @ 265 Reps** **265 x 70% = 185.5 Reps (Low Effort Intensity)** **265 x 80% = 212 Reps (High Effort Intensity)**
Example:	**Running Max Distance Benchmark Number @ 800 Meters** **800 x 70% = 560 Meters (Low Effort Intensity)** **800 x 80% = 640 Meters (High Effort Intensity)**

24-Day Effort Intensity and Rotation Schedule:

Day 1	**@ Max Effort/Baseline**
Day 2	**@66% to 70% of Max Effort**
Day 3	**@76% to 80% of Max Effort**
Rotate Order	
Day 4	**@ Max Effort/Benchmark**
Day 5	**@66% to 70% of Max Effort**
Day 6	**@76% to 80% of Max Effort**
Rotate Order	
Day 7	**@ Max Effort/Benchmark**
Day 8	**@66% to 70% of Max Effort**
Day 9	**@76% to 80% of Max Effort**
Rotate Order	
Day 10	**@ Max Effort/Benchmark**
Day 11	**@66% to 70% of Max Effort**
Day 12	**@76% to 80% of Max Effort**
Rotate Order	
Day 13	**@ Max Effort/Benchmark**
Day 14	**@66% to 70% of Max Effort**
Day 15	**@76% to 80% of Max Effort**
Rotate Order	
Day 16	**@ Max Effort/Benchmark**
Day 17	**@66% to 70% of Max Effort**
Day 18	**@76% to 80% of Max Effort**
Rotate Order	
Day 19	**@ Max Effort/Benchmark**
Day 20	**@66% to 70% of Max Effort**
Day 21	**@76% to 80% of Max Effort**
Rotate Order	
Day 22	**@ Max Effort/Benchmark**
Day 23	**@66% to 70% of Max Effort**
Day 24	**@76% to 80% of Max Effort**

Establish Specific Isolated Thresholds of Cardiovascular (HrMx), Anaerobic (Vo2 Max), and Muscular Endurance (m.e.t.).

Review Your 24-Day Training Plan Notes and Compare Initial Benchmark Data Final Results. You will find that Muscular Endurance Increased while Post Exercise Heart Rates Decreased as the Body Became more Efficient.

***See the Evolution of Fitness? ***

*Note:

When I teach someone the 24-Day plan and have done so successfully 100% of the time since 2018, the very first thing I do is to find a person's physical strengths and weaknesses. The first important thing is to choose the desired amount of exercise intervals. Most choose between 4 and 8.

Everyone has strengths and weaknesses, but at the end of my programs, instead of calling them strengths and weaknesses, a person can call themselves Cross Exercise Efficient.*

On day one in the order of Exercises chosen:

The "Baseline" Max Effort Rep volume is required to show your beginning fitness level. Here is why:

Every third day after that first day requires you to push the body at 100% Effort Max Rep volume, succeed in hitting the Baseline and push harder to exceed a new benchmark.

Here is what happens physiologically and psychologically when a person actually sees their max heart rate lower while at the same time their max Rep volume increases every 3rd day....**it's a giant morale confidence booster** (psychology 101), and seeing the evolution of their fitness level improving right in front of them...wow...it's fun to watch. When they run up to me and tell me how they did...**that's the reward**!

> **"One must know his or her Baseline Cross Exercise Efficiency Strengths and Weaknesses before one can create Benchmark Capabilities Within their Individual Fitness Evolution."**
> **Heathen Warrior**

Section 8:

Miscellaneous List of Exercises

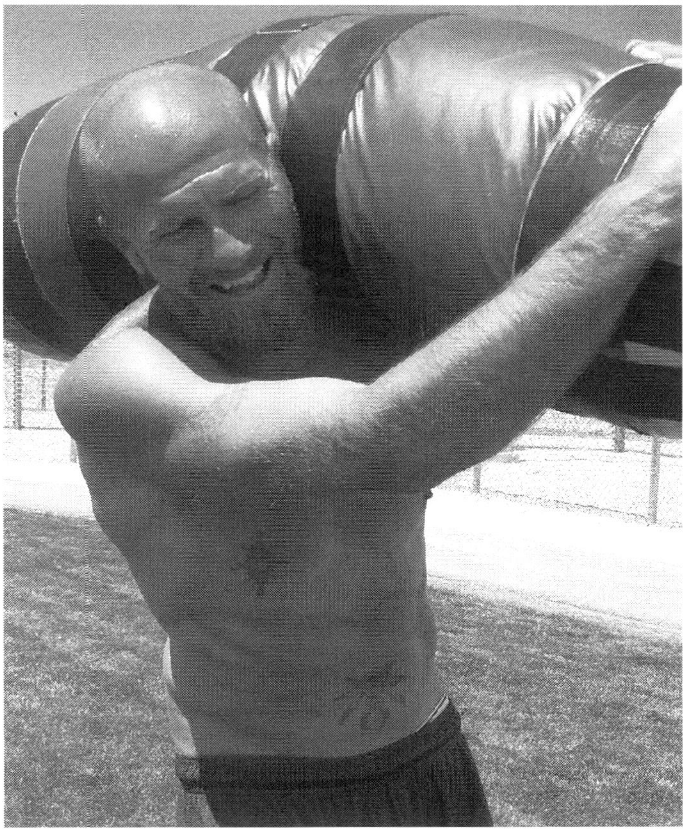

Miscellaneous List of Exercises:

A. Maximum High Effort Intensity Exercises
&
B. Combination Exercises (Multiple Exercises Per Round as Rep/Set)

1. Ana/Vo2 Cardio Intervals (Av^2/ci)
2. Anaerobic/Vo2 Cross-Exercise Muscular Endurance-Max Cardio And Recovery Interval Training (Av^2/ceme-mc and rit)
3. Max Intensity Interval Training (M.I.I.T.)
4. High-Intensity Interval Training (H.I.I.T.)

C. Low Effort Intensity/Low Impact Exercises

1. Recovery Training
2. Low-Intensity Interval Training (L.I.I.T.)

D. Static/Dynamic Instructions and Exercise Routines
E. Free Weight Exercises (When Available)

A. Maximum Intensity and High Effort Intensity Exercises:

Anaerobic
Vo2
Cardio
Muscular Endurance Threshold

No Free Weight Available

Single Element Sample Exercises:

Running
Stair Incline Running
Hill sprint Running
Box Jumps (24" to 48")
Double Under Jump Rope
Rowing Machine (Concept 2)
Muscle-ups (Front/Reverse Grip)
DeadStop Burpee Jumps
Toes To Bar
Jump Lunges
Jump Squats
Cycle (Airdyne)

Apply a blend of these Exercise for:
Max/High-Intensity Interval Training (M.I.I.T./H.I.I.T.)

B. Combination Max Intensity

Free Weight Not Available
Double and Triple Element Sample Exercises:

Examples:

Run 100 to 400 Meters with 1-5 Exercise Reps of:

Muscle-ups
Toes to Bar
Kipping Handstand Push-ups
DeadStop Burpee Jumps
Box Jumps (24" to 48")
Static/Dynamic Routines

Run 1000 to 5000 Meters with 1-10 Exercise Reps of:

Jump Lunges
Rowing Machine
Cycle (Airdyne)
Jump Squats
Double Under Jump Rope
Av^2/ci

10 to 30-Minute Workouts of "As Many Reps As Possible.":
1 Rep = 1 DeadStop Burpee Jump and 1 Muscle-up

Examples:

DeadStop Burpee Jump and Muscle-up
Reverse Grip Muscle-Up and Toes to Bar
DeadStop Burpee Jump and Box Jump

*The DeadStop phase of the Burpee means that Bodyweight is completely released at the bottom of the push-up by raising both hands from the ground before standing up to complete the Burpee Exercise: "DeadStop Burpee Jump" *

C. Low Effort Intensity/ Low Impact Exercises:

Low-Intensity Interval Training (L.I.I.T.)
Recovery Training

Sample Exercises:

Low Effort Intensity Tempo Running	**Jumping Jacks**
Low-Intensity Walking	**Bridge**
Plank (Static)	**Push-ups**
Plank Mountain Climbers (Dynamic)	**Sit-ups**
Side Plank (Static)	**Runners Lunge (Static)**
Side Plank Crunches (Dynamic)	**Static Handstand**
Jump Rope Single Under	**Pull-ups**
Runners Lunge Crunches (Dynamic)	**Mountain Climbers**
Bicycle Crunches/Horizontal	**Back Extensions**
Ab Extensions	**Swimming**
Stationary Cycle/Bike Riding	

Examples:

- Run Easy Temp for 400 – 800 Meters with 1 to 20 Exercise Reps @ Low Effort Intensity/ Level 3 Zones 1-3 For 10 to 30 Minutes of:
- Low-Intensity Interval Training (L.I.I.T.)
- *Use Sample Exercises*
- Walk for 30 to 60 Minutes
- Cycle (Stationary) or a Standard Bike Ride for 30 to 60 Minutes at Easy Tempo Pace.
- Swim for 30 Minutes mixed with Treading Water and Power Walking at Waist Deep Water Level.

Rule of Recovery Exercises Routines

Low Effort Intensity Cross Exercises
50 to 75% of Max Heart Rate Training Range

Low-Intensity impact on:

Muscular System
Cardiovascular System
Pulmonary/Aerobic System
Skeletal System (Bones and Joints)

D. Static/Dynamic Instructions Exercise Routines:

Static/Dynamic
This Exercise routine is unique and versatile. It can be applied to any Exercise that is performed safely, holding body weight, free weight, or resistance bands comfortably when at a static muscle contraction and then executing the Rep(s) in good form dynamically.
The Static Phase of the Exercise means "Hold" the Position of Muscle contraction.
Dynamic Phase of the Exercise Means "Perform" the Exercise Rep(s) Dictated by Static Count.

***Exercise Rep Ascend" Means UP (1-5) ***
***Exercise Rep Descend" means DOWN (5-1) ***

Example:

5-1 Static/Dynamic Routine of Push-ups as Follows
Rep(s)/Set Descend

1st SET	**Assume the Top of Push-up Position. Hold that position for a Full 5 Second Count Static Then Immediately Perform 5 Reps without Stopping. Continue Descending to One Second Static/One Rep Dynamic**
2nd SET	**4 Second Static Hold and 4 Reps Dynamic**
3rd SET	**3 Second Static Hold and 3 Reps Dynamic**
4th SET	**2 Second Static Hold and 2 Reps Dynamic**
5th SET	**1 Second Static Hold and 1 Rep Dynamic**

Rep Ascend and Rep Ascend/Descend Pyramid Routines:

Rep Ascend Routine	Total Reps	Rep Ascend/Descend Pyramid Routine	Total Reps
1-2	3	1-2/2-1	6
1-3	6	1-3/3-1	12
1-4	10	1-4/4-1	20
1-5	15	1-5/5-1	30
1-6	21	1-6/6-1	42
1-7	28	1-7/7-1	56
1-8	36	1-8/8-1	72
1-9	45	1-9/9-1	90
1-10	55	1-10/10-1	110

Example Exercises for Static/Dynamic Routines:

Shoulder Presses (Free Weight)	Pull-ups (Wide and Close Grip)
Upright Rows (Free Weight)	Chin-ups (Wide and Close Grip)
Shoulder Shrugs (Free Weight)	Body Squats
Lateral Rows (Free Weight)	Lunges
Bench Press (Free Weight)	Handstand Push-ups
Squats (Free Weight)	Push-ups
Bicep Curls (Free Weight)	Sit-ups
Tricep Extensions (Free Weight)	Dips
Clean Press (Free Weight)	Mountain Climbers
Dead Lift (Free Weight)	Even Muscle-ups

Choose the Rep/Set that meets your Current Fitness Level… Then, ELEVATE THE INTENSITY FOR UNLIMITED PROGRESS!

E. Free Weight Exercises

When Available

Squat Thrusters
Clean and Press
Squat
Dead Lifts
Overhead Snatch
Dumbbell Snatch
Bench Press
Jerk Clean
Weighted Lateral Rows
Medicine Ball Squats

Apply Free Weight Exercises to the Examples in Section 8 Part B for Individual Training Needs

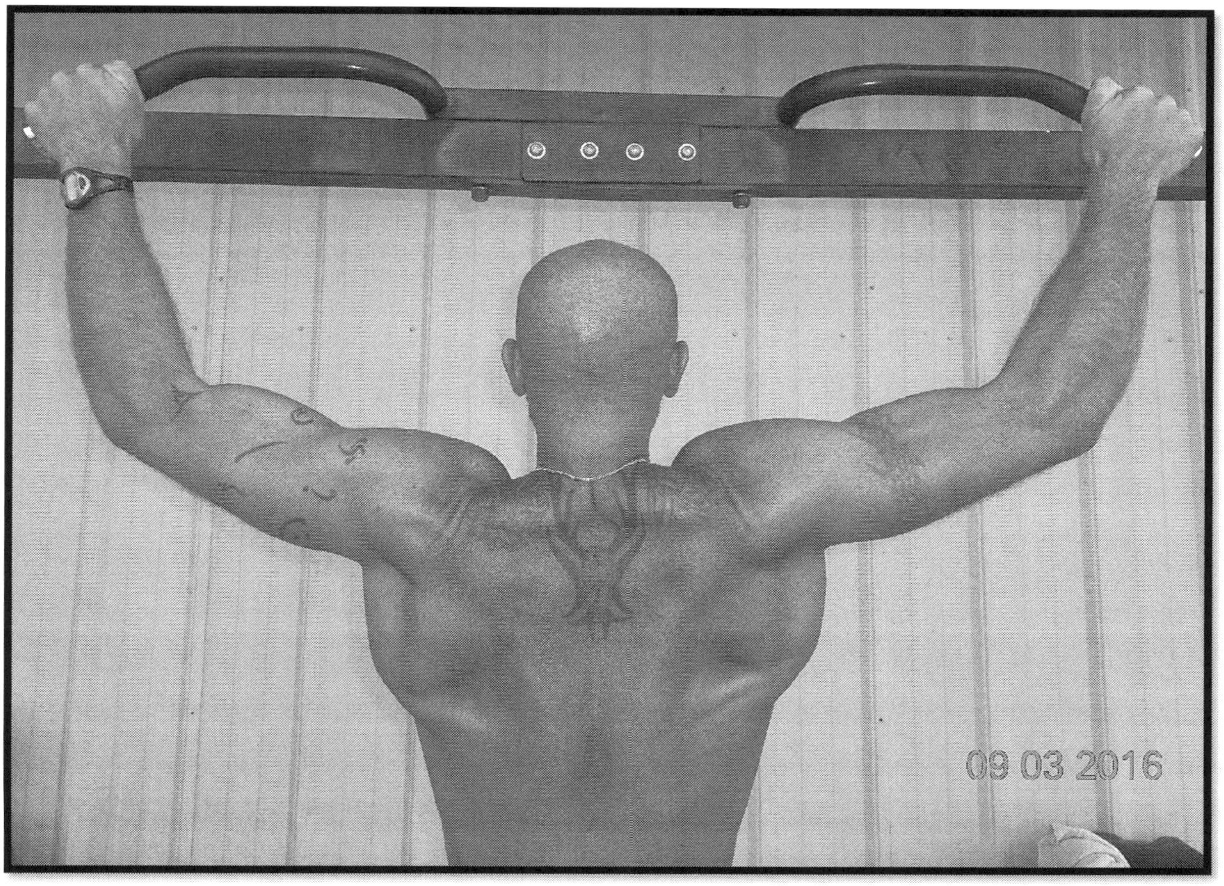

NEVER SACRIFICE SAFE EXERCISE FORM FOR A Rep!

Most injuries occur when the primary connective tissue is compromised during muscle failure and fatigue.

Actively evaluate your mechanical form during Exercises. Be honest with your performance when training to complete exhaustion. When your form feels sloppy, Step Back and take three Deep Breaths, Compose Yourself, Perform a Rep, and Repeat the Process as Necessary.

Continue to Evaluate safe Exercise Form, Breathing, and Heart Rate Management.

Heathen Warrior Demon Burpee's

Demonz Burpee's Lineup Av²/10x-ci Demonz Multi Movement Exercises	
1. DMZ 1/j-jax	6. DMZ p-rottz/vbc
2. DMZ jmp-in/j-jax	7. DMZ sprtn/jmp
3. DMZ lp-sk/smc/ots	8. DMZ t2/j-jax
4. DMZ spc/vbc	9. DMZ rlc/otrl
5. DMZ t2/jmp-in/vbc	10. *7 Step Heathen Demon Burpee
Description Below	

Primary Element of Demonz:

~Dead Stop Push-ups~

Secondary Element (s):

(with exercise acronyms)

jumping jax (j-jax)	vertical bicycle crunches (vbc)
overhead towel squats (ots)	overhead towel reverse lunges (otrl)
runners lunge crunches (rlc)	side plank crunches (spc)
jump in (jmp-in)	plank mountain climbers (pmc)
standard mountain climbers(smc)	left-right t2-push-ups (t2)
arm jax high knee kicks (j-jax/hkk)	spartan jump (sprtn-jmp)
(left-right) plank rotations (p-rottz)	low push-up side kick (lp-sk)
DeadStop burpees (dmz/demonz)	

7 Step Heathen Demon Burpee

1	DeadStop push-up with jump in/jump-out
2	(left-right) low push-up side kick
3	(left-right) side plank crunches
4	(left-right) dead stop t2-push-ups
5	(left-right) runners lunge crunches
6	standard mountain climber
7	a. overhead towel squat b. (left-right) high knee kick c. (left-right)overhead towel reverse lunge

Section 9:

Glossary

of

Terminology

Common Acronyms Used in this Manual

A.L.O.I.	=	Average Level Of Intensity
Av^2/ceme-mc and rit	=	Anaerobic Vo2/Cross-Exercise Muscular Endurance-Max Cardio And Recovery Interval Training
Av^2/ci	=	Anaerobic Vo2 cardio intervals
BMI	=	Body mass index
BPM	=	Beats Per Minute
C.E.E.	=	Cross Exercise Efficient
C.E.P.S.	=	Cross Exercise Pyramid Set
C.E.R.A.C.	=	Cross Exercise Rep Ascension Circuit
H.I.I.T.	=	High-Intensity Interval Training
HR	=	Heart Rate
HvI	=	Hybrid VO2 Intervals
KCal	=	Calorie
Km K kilometer	=	Kilometer (1000 Meters) (1000 Meters = .6214 Miles) (1000 Meters = 1093.664 Yards)
L.I.I.T.	=	Low-Intensity Interval Training
LPS or lps	=	Laps
M.I.I.T.	=	Max Intensity Interval Training
MI or mi	=	Mile (1760 yards) (1760 yards = 1609.344 Meters) (1760 Yards= 5280 Feet)
MxHr or HrMx	=	Max Heart Rate
NR-10.8	=	No Run-10.8
N.S.R.G.	=	Non-Standard Reverse Grip
PB	=	Personal Best
PBM	=	Personal Benchmark
P.O.P.O.	=	Percentage of Physical Output
Repetition	=	Repeating an Exercise Interval
Reps	=	Exercise Rep
Rep^2/squared	=	Reps Multiplied by Variable
PR	=	Personal Record
RNDS or rnds	=	Rounds
S.F.G.	=	Standard Front Grip
Vo2 Max	=	Maximal Oxygen Uptake
WOD or W.O.D.	=	Work out of the day
WR-10	=	With Run-10

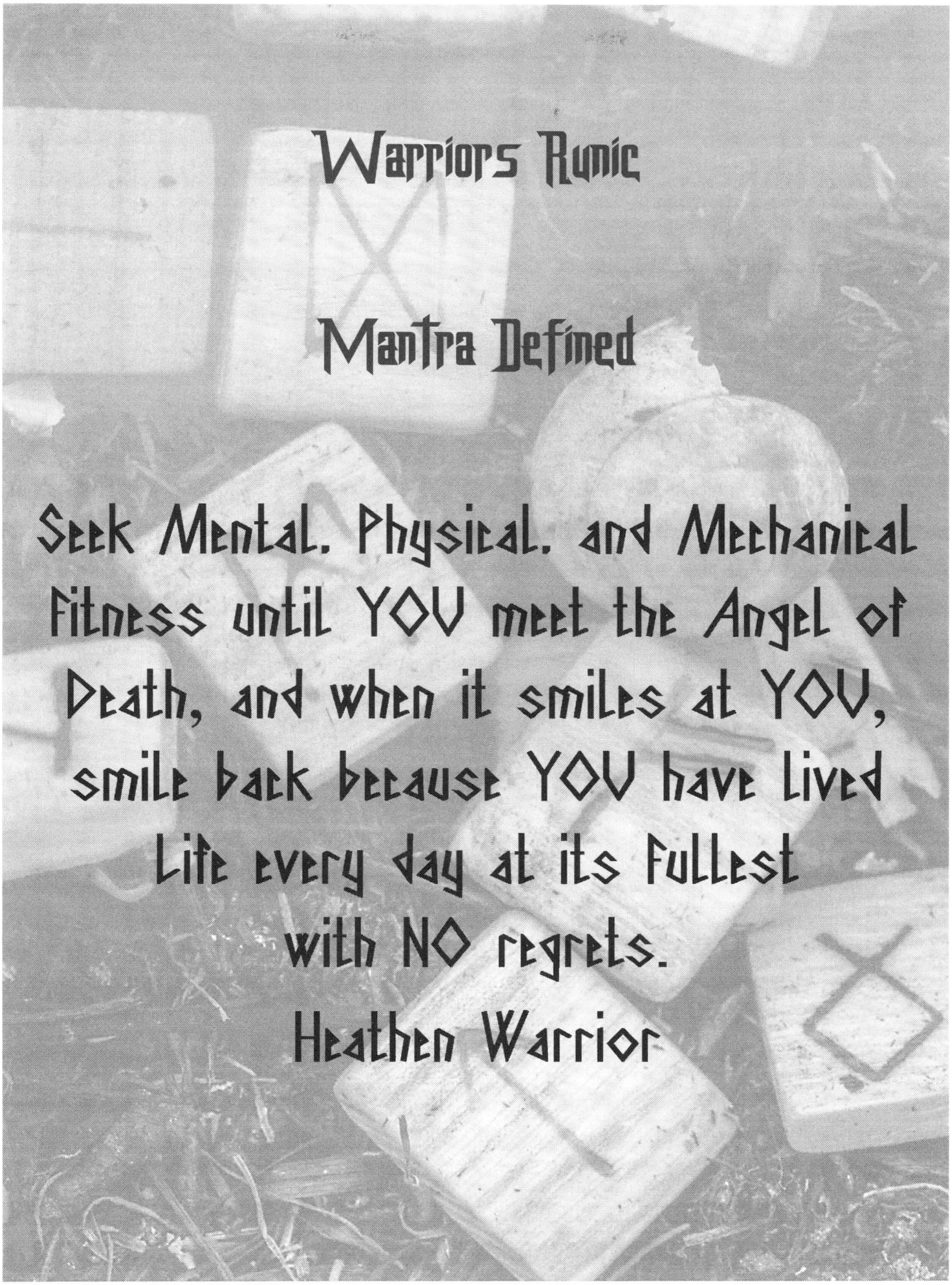

Warriors Runic

Mantra Defined

Seek Mental, Physical, and Mechanical Fitness until YOU meet the Angel of Death, and when it smiles at YOU, smile back because YOU have lived life every day at its fullest with NO regrets.

Heathen Warrior

Calendar Log and

Training Data Section

Features:

- 2-Year Calendar Log
- Av^2/ci WOD sheets
- Progress Notes for Documenting Your Fitness Evolution
- Blank Lined Paper for your Writing needs

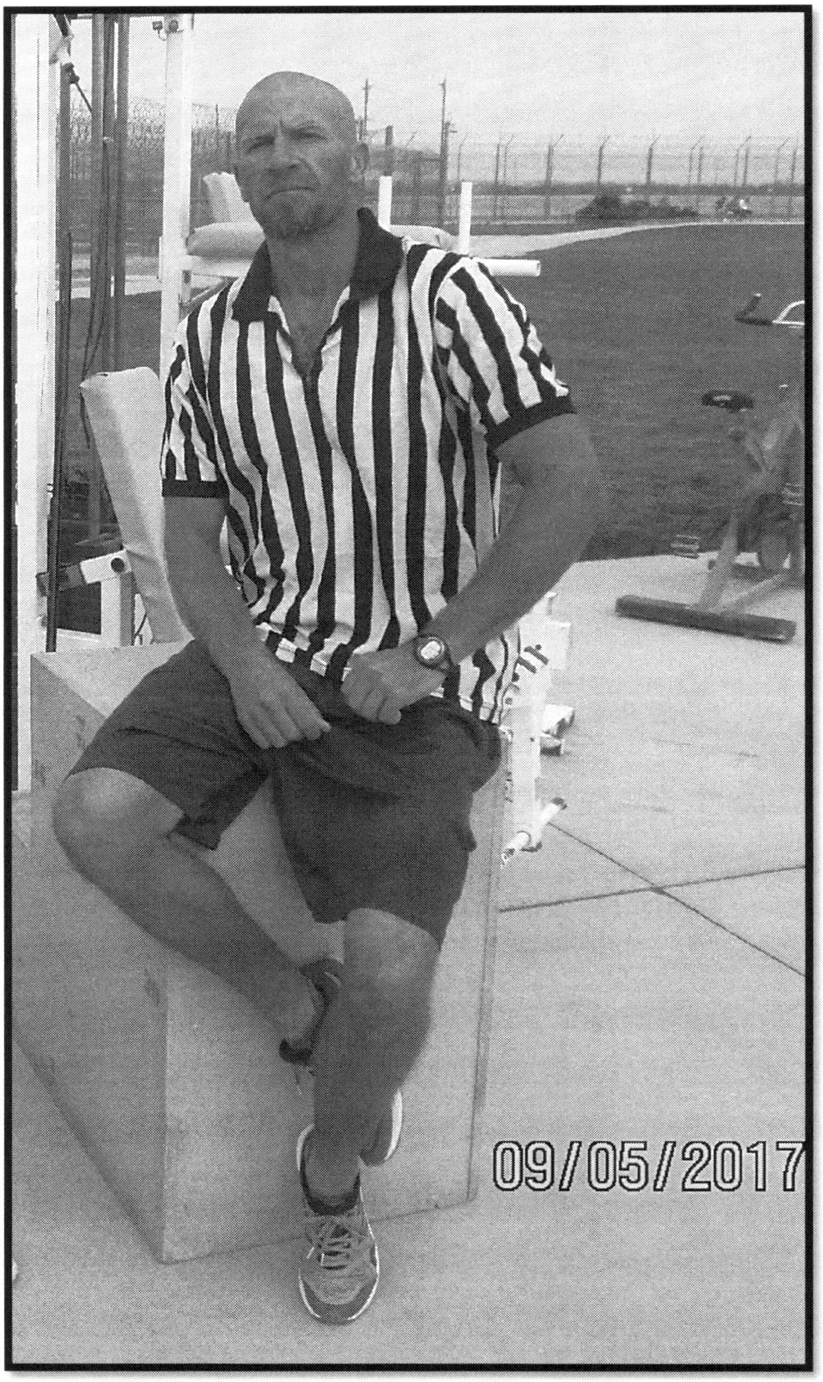
09/05/2017

6 Week Training Calendar
Month Year

SUNDAY	MONDAY	TUESDAY	WEDNESDAY	THURSDAY	FRIDAY	SATURDAY

Week 1

Date:	Date:	Date:	Date:	Date:	Date:	Date:
Mileage:	Mileage:	Mileage:	Mileage:	Mileage:	Mileage:	Mileage:

Week 2

Date:	Date:	Date:	Date:	Date:	Date:	Date:
Mileage:	Mileage:	Mileage:	Mileage:	Mileage:	Mileage:	Mileage:

Week 3

Date:	Date:	Date:	Date:	Date:	Date:	Date:
Mileage:	Mileage:	Mileage:	Mileage:	Mileage:	Mileage:	Mileage:

Week 4

Date:	Date:	Date:	Date:	Date:	Date:	Date:
Mileage:	Mileage:	Mileage:	Mileage:	Mileage:	Mileage:	Mileage:

Week 5

Date:	Date:	Date:	Date:	Date:	Date:	Date:
Mileage:	Mileage:	Mileage:	Mileage:	Mileage:	Mileage:	Mileage:

Week 6

Date:	Date:	Date:	Date:	Date:	Date:	Date:
Mileage:	Mileage:	Mileage:	Mileage:	Mileage:	Mileage:	Mileage:

Ana/Vo2 CARDIO INTERVALS
(Hvi's) mcw est. '13

	Date:	am or pm	Intervals:
	W.O.D.:	rps/rnds/lps	HrMx%
1			
2			
3			
4			
5			
6			
7			
8			
9			
10			
11			
12			
		A.L.O.I @:	

Ana/Vo2 CARDIO INTERVALS
(Hvi's) mcw est. '13

	Date:	am or pm	Intervals:
	W.O.D.:	rps/rnds/lps	HrMx%
1			
2			
3			
4			
5			
6			
7			
8			
9			
10			
11			
12			
		A.L.O.I @:	

Ana/Vo2 CARDIO INTERVALS
(Hvi's) mcw est. '13

	Date:	am or pm	Intervals:
	W.O.D.:	rps/rnds/lps	HrMx%
1			
2			
3			
4			
5			
6			
7			
8			
9			
10			
11			
12			
		A.L.O.I @:	

Ana/Vo2 CARDIO INTERVALS
(Hvi's) mcw est. '13

	Date:	am or pm	Intervals:
	W.O.D.:	rps/rnds/lps	HrMx%
1			
2			
3			
4			
5			
6			
7			
8			
9			
10			
11			
12			
		A.L.O.I @:	

Ana/Vo2 CARDIO INTERVALS
(Hvi's) mcw est. '13

	Date:	am or pm	Intervals:
	W.O.D.:	rps/rnds/lps	HrMx%
1			
2			
3			
4			
5			
6			
7			
8			
9			
10			
11			
12			
		A.L.O.I @:	

Ana/Vo2 CARDIO INTERVALS
(Hvi's) mcw est. '13

	Date:	am or pm	Intervals:
	W.O.D.:	rps/rnds/lps	HrMx%
1			
2			
3			
4			
5			
6			
7			
8			
9			
10			
11			
12			
		A.L.O.I @:	

Ana/Vo2 CARDIO INTERVALS

(Hvi's) mcw est. '13

Date:	am or pm	Intervals:
W.O.D.:	rps/rnds/lps	HrMx%
1		
2		
3		
4		
5		
6		
7		
8		
9		
10		
11		
12		
	A.L.O.I @:	

Ana/Vo2 CARDIO INTERVALS

(Hvi's) mcw est. '13

Date:	am or pm	Intervals:
W.O.D.:	rps/rnds/lps	HrMx%
1		
2		
3		
4		
5		
6		
7		
8		
9		
10		
11		
12		
	A.L.O.I @:	

Ana/Vo2 CARDIO INTERVALS

(Hvi's) mcw est. '13

Date:	am or pm	Intervals:
W.O.D.:	rps/rnds/lps	HrMx%
1		
2		
3		
4		
5		
6		
7		
8		
9		
10		
11		
12		
	A.L.O.I @:	

Ana/Vo2 CARDIO INTERVALS

(Hvi's) mcw est. '13

Date:	am or pm	Intervals:
W.O.D.:	rps/rnds/lps	HrMx%
1		
2		
3		
4		
5		
6		
7		
8		
9		
10		
11		
12		
	A.L.O.I @:	

Ana/Vo2 CARDIO INTERVALS

(Hvi's) mcw est. '13

Date:	am or pm	Intervals:
W.O.D.:	rps/rnds/lps	HrMx%
1		
2		
3		
4		
5		
6		
7		
8		
9		
10		
11		
12		
	A.L.O.I @:	

Ana/Vo2 CARDIO INTERVALS

(Hvi's) mcw est. '13

Date:	am or pm	Intervals:
W.O.D.:	rps/rnds/lps	HrMx%
1		
2		
3		
4		
5		
6		
7		
8		
9		
10		
11		
12		
	A.L.O.I @:	

Ana/Vo2 CARDIO INTERVALS
(Hvi's) mcw est. '13

	Date:	am or pm	Intervals:
	W.O.D.:	rps/rnds/lps	HrMx%
1			
2			
3			
4			
5			
6			
7			
8			
9			
10			
11			
12			
		A.L.O.I @:	

Ana/Vo2 CARDIO INTERVALS
(Hvi's) mcw est. '13

	Date:	am or pm	Intervals:
	W.O.D.:	rps/rnds/lps	HrMx%
1			
2			
3			
4			
5			
6			
7			
8			
9			
10			
11			
12			
		A.L.O.I @:	

Ana/Vo2 CARDIO INTERVALS
(Hvi's) mcw est. '13

	Date:	am or pm	Intervals:
	W.O.D.:	rps/rnds/lps	HrMx%
1			
2			
3			
4			
5			
6			
7			
8			
9			
10			
11			
12			
		A.L.O.I @:	

Ana/Vo2 CARDIO INTERVALS
(Hvi's) mcw est. '13

	Date:	am or pm	Intervals:
	W.O.D.:	rps/rnds/lps	HrMx%
1			
2			
3			
4			
5			
6			
7			
8			
9			
10			
11			
12			
		A.L.O.I @:	

Ana/Vo2 CARDIO INTERVALS
(Hvi's) mcw est. '13

	Date:	am or pm	Intervals:
	W.O.D.:	rps/rnds/lps	HrMx%
1			
2			
3			
4			
5			
6			
7			
8			
9			
10			
11			
12			
		A.L.O.I @:	

Ana/Vo2 CARDIO INTERVALS
(Hvi's) mcw est. '13

	Date:	am or pm	Intervals:
	W.O.D.:	rps/rnds/lps	HrMx%
1			
2			
3			
4			
5			
6			
7			
8			
9			
10			
11			
12			
		A.L.O.I @:	

Ana/Vo2 CARDIO INTERVALS
(Hvi's) mcw est. '13

	Date:	am or pm	Intervals:
	W.O.D.:	rps/rnds/lps	HrMx%
1			
2			
3			
4			
5			
6			
7			
8			
9			
10			
11			
12			
		A.L.O.I @:	

Ana/Vo2 CARDIO INTERVALS
(Hvi's) mcw est. '13

	Date:	am or pm	Intervals:
	W.O.D.:	rps/rnds/lps	HrMx%
1			
2			
3			
4			
5			
6			
7			
8			
9			
10			
11			
12			
		A.L.O.I @:	

Ana/Vo2 CARDIO INTERVALS
(Hvi's) mcw est. '13

	Date:	am or pm	Intervals:
	W.O.D.:	rps/rnds/lps	HrMx%
1			
2			
3			
4			
5			
6			
7			
8			
9			
10			
11			
12			
		A.L.O.I @:	

Ana/Vo2 CARDIO INTERVALS
(Hvi's) mcw est. '13

	Date:	am or pm	Intervals:
	W.O.D.:	rps/rnds/lps	HrMx%
1			
2			
3			
4			
5			
6			
7			
8			
9			
10			
11			
12			
		A.L.O.I @:	

Ana/Vo2 CARDIO INTERVALS
(Hvi's) mcw est. '13

	Date:	am or pm	Intervals:
	W.O.D.:	rps/rnds/lps	HrMx%
1			
2			
3			
4			
5			
6			
7			
8			
9			
10			
11			
12			
		A.L.O.I @:	

Ana/Vo2 CARDIO INTERVALS
(Hvi's) mcw est. '13

	Date:	am or pm	Intervals:
	W.O.D.:	rps/rnds/lps	HrMx%
1			
2			
3			
4			
5			
6			
7			
8			
9			
10			
11			
12			
		A.L.O.I @:	

Ana/Vo2 CARDIO INTERVALS

(Hvi's) mcw est. '13

	Date:	am or pm	Intervals:
	W.O.D.:	rps/rnds/lps	HrMx%
1			
2			
3			
4			
5			
6			
7			
8			
9			
10			
11			
12			
		A.L.O.I @:	

Ana/Vo2 CARDIO INTERVALS

(Hvi's) mcw est. '13

	Date:	am or pm	Intervals:
	W.O.D.:	rps/rnds/lps	HrMx%
1			
2			
3			
4			
5			
6			
7			
8			
9			
10			
11			
12			
		A.L.O.I @:	

Ana/Vo2 CARDIO INTERVALS

(Hvi's) mcw est. '13

	Date:	am or pm	Intervals:
	W.O.D.:	rps/rnds/lps	HrMx%
1			
2			
3			
4			
5			
6			
7			
8			
9			
10			
11			
12			
		A.L.O.I @:	

Ana/Vo2 CARDIO INTERVALS

(Hvi's) mcw est. '13

	Date:	am or pm	Intervals:
	W.O.D.:	rps/rnds/lps	HrMx%
1			
2			
3			
4			
5			
6			
7			
8			
9			
10			
11			
12			
		A.L.O.I @:	

Ana/Vo2 CARDIO INTERVALS

(Hvi's) mcw est. '13

	Date:	am or pm	Intervals:
	W.O.D.:	rps/rnds/lps	HrMx%
1			
2			
3			
4			
5			
6			
7			
8			
9			
10			
11			
12			
		A.L.O.I @:	

Ana/Vo2 CARDIO INTERVALS

(Hvi's) mcw est. '13

	Date:	am or pm	Intervals:
	W.O.D.:	rps/rnds/lps	HrMx%
1			
2			
3			
4			
5			
6			
7			
8			
9			
10			
11			
12			
		A.L.O.I @:	

FITNESS EVOLUTION NOTES:

Track your Training Effort Intensity Level Zones, Calorie Expense, and Personal Benchmark Record Data

DATE:__________ DATA:	DATE:__________ DATA:
DATE:__________ DATA:	DATE:__________ DATA:
DATE:__________ DATA:	DATE:__________ DATA:
DATE:__________ DATA:	DATE:__________ DATA:
DATE:__________ DATA:	DATE:__________ DATA:
DATE:__________ DATA:	DATE:__________ DATA:
DATE:__________ DATA:	DATE:__________ DATA:

FITNESS EVOLUTION NOTES:

Track your Training Effort Intensity Level Zones, Calorie Expense, and Personal Benchmark Record Data

DATE: DATA:	DATE: DATA:
DATE: DATA:	DATE: DATA:
DATE: DATA:	DATE: DATA:
DATE: DATA:	DATE: DATA:
DATE: DATA:	DATE: DATA:
DATE: DATA:	DATE: DATA:
DATE: DATA:	DATE: DATA:

NOTES:

NOTES:

6 Week Training Calendar
Month Year

SUNDAY	MONDAY	TUESDAY	WEDNESDAY	THURSDAY	FRIDAY	SATURDAY

Week 1

Date:	Date:	Date:	Date:	Date:	Date:	Date:
Mileage:	Mileage:	Mileage:	Mileage:	Mileage:	Mileage:	Mileage:

Week 2

Date:	Date:	Date:	Date:	Date:	Date:	Date:
Mileage:	Mileage:	Mileage:	Mileage:	Mileage:	Mileage:	Mileage:

Week 3

Date:	Date:	Date:	Date:	Date:	Date:	Date:
Mileage:	Mileage:	Mileage:	Mileage:	Mileage:	Mileage:	Mileage:

Week 4

Date:	Date:	Date:	Date:	Date:	Date:	Date:
Mileage:	Mileage:	Mileage:	Mileage:	Mileage:	Mileage:	Mileage:

Week 5

Date:	Date:	Date:	Date:	Date:	Date:	Date:
Mileage:	Mileage:	Mileage:	Mileage:	Mileage:	Mileage:	Mileage:

Week 6

Date:	Date:	Date:	Date:	Date:	Date:	Date:
Mileage:	Mileage:	Mileage:	Mileage:	Mileage:	Mileage:	Mileage:

Ana/Vo2 CARDIO INTERVALS

(Hvi's) mcw est. '13

	Date:	am or pm	Intervals:
	W.O.D.:	rps/rnds/lps	HrMx%
1			
2			
3			
4			
5			
6			
7			
8			
9			
10			
11			
12			
		A.L.O.I @:	

Ana/Vo2 CARDIO INTERVALS

(Hvi's) mcw est. '13

	Date:	am or pm	Intervals:
	W.O.D.:	rps/rnds/lps	HrMx%
1			
2			
3			
4			
5			
6			
7			
8			
9			
10			
11			
12			
		A.L.O.I @:	

Ana/Vo2 CARDIO INTERVALS

(Hvi's) mcw est. '13

	Date:	am or pm	Intervals:
	W.O.D.:	rps/rnds/lps	HrMx%
1			
2			
3			
4			
5			
6			
7			
8			
9			
10			
11			
12			
		A.L.O.I @:	

Ana/Vo2 CARDIO INTERVALS

(Hvi's) mcw est. '13

	Date:	am or pm	Intervals:
	W.O.D.:	rps/rnds/lps	HrMx%
1			
2			
3			
4			
5			
6			
7			
8			
9			
10			
11			
12			
		A.L.O.I @:	

Ana/Vo2 CARDIO INTERVALS

(Hvi's) mcw est. '13

	Date:	am or pm	Intervals:
	W.O.D.:	rps/rnds/lps	HrMx%
1			
2			
3			
4			
5			
6			
7			
8			
9			
10			
11			
12			
		A.L.O.I @:	

Ana/Vo2 CARDIO INTERVALS

(Hvi's) mcw est. '13

	Date:	am or pm	Intervals:
	W.O.D.:	rps/rnds/lps	HrMx%
1			
2			
3			
4			
5			
6			
7			
8			
9			
10			
11			
12			
		A.L.O.I @:	

Ana/Vo2 CARDIO INTERVALS

(Hvi's) mcw est. '13

	Date:	am or pm	Intervals:
	W.O.D.:	rps/rnds/lps	HrMx%
1			
2			
3			
4			
5			
6			
7			
8			
9			
10			
11			
12			
		A.L.O.I @:	

Ana/Vo2 CARDIO INTERVALS

(Hvi's) mcw est. '13

	Date:	am or pm	Intervals:
	W.O.D.:	rps/rnds/lps	HrMx%
1			
2			
3			
4			
5			
6			
7			
8			
9			
10			
11			
12			
		A.L.O.I @:	

Ana/Vo2 CARDIO INTERVALS

(Hvi's) mcw est. '13

	Date:	am or pm	Intervals:
	W.O.D.:	rps/rnds/lps	HrMx%
1			
2			
3			
4			
5			
6			
7			
8			
9			
10			
11			
12			
		A.L.O.I @:	

Ana/Vo2 CARDIO INTERVALS

(Hvi's) mcw est. '13

	Date:	am or pm	Intervals:
	W.O.D.:	rps/rnds/lps	HrMx%
1			
2			
3			
4			
5			
6			
7			
8			
9			
10			
11			
12			
		A.L.O.I @:	

Ana/Vo2 CARDIO INTERVALS

(Hvi's) mcw est. '13

	Date:	am or pm	Intervals:
	W.O.D.:	rps/rnds/lps	HrMx%
1			
2			
3			
4			
5			
6			
7			
8			
9			
10			
11			
12			
		A.L.O.I @:	

Ana/Vo2 CARDIO INTERVALS

(Hvi's) mcw est. '13

	Date:	am or pm	Intervals:
	W.O.D.:	rps/rnds/lps	HrMx%
1			
2			
3			
4			
5			
6			
7			
8			
9			
10			
11			
12			
		A.L.O.I @:	

Ana/Vo2 CARDIO INTERVALS
(Hvi's) mcw est. '13

	Date:	am or pm	Intervals:
	W.O.D.:	rps/rnds/lps	HrMx%
1			
2			
3			
4			
5			
6			
7			
8			
9			
10			
11			
12			
		A.L.O.I @:	

Ana/Vo2 CARDIO INTERVALS
(Hvi's) mcw est. '13

	Date:	am or pm	Intervals:
	W.O.D.:	rps/rnds/lps	HrMx%
1			
2			
3			
4			
5			
6			
7			
8			
9			
10			
11			
12			
		A.L.O.I @:	

Ana/Vo2 CARDIO INTERVALS
(Hvi's) mcw est. '13

	Date:	am or pm	Intervals:
	W.O.D.:	rps/rnds/lps	HrMx%
1			
2			
3			
4			
5			
6			
7			
8			
9			
10			
11			
12			
		A.L.O.I @:	

Ana/Vo2 CARDIO INTERVALS
(Hvi's) mcw est. '13

	Date:	am or pm	Intervals:
	W.O.D.:	rps/rnds/lps	HrMx%
1			
2			
3			
4			
5			
6			
7			
8			
9			
10			
11			
12			
		A.L.O.I @:	

Ana/Vo2 CARDIO INTERVALS
(Hvi's) mcw est. '13

	Date:	am or pm	Intervals:
	W.O.D.:	rps/rnds/lps	HrMx%
1			
2			
3			
4			
5			
6			
7			
8			
9			
10			
11			
12			
		A.L.O.I @:	

Ana/Vo2 CARDIO INTERVALS
(Hvi's) mcw est. '13

	Date:	am or pm	Intervals:
	W.O.D.:	rps/rnds/lps	HrMx%
1			
2			
3			
4			
5			
6			
7			
8			
9			
10			
11			
12			
		A.L.O.I @:	

Ana/Vo2 CARDIO INTERVALS
(Hvi's) mcw est. '13

	Date:	am or pm	Intervals:
	W.O.D.:	rps/rnds/lps	HrMx%
1			
2			
3			
4			
5			
6			
7			
8			
9			
10			
11			
12			
		A.L.O.I @:	

Ana/Vo2 CARDIO INTERVALS
(Hvi's) mcw est. '13

	Date:	am or pm	Intervals:
	W.O.D.:	rps/rnds/lps	HrMx%
1			
2			
3			
4			
5			
6			
7			
8			
9			
10			
11			
12			
		A.L.O.I @:	

Ana/Vo2 CARDIO INTERVALS
(Hvi's) mcw est. '13

	Date:	am or pm	Intervals:
	W.O.D.:	rps/rnds/lps	HrMx%
1			
2			
3			
4			
5			
6			
7			
8			
9			
10			
11			
12			
		A.L.O.I @:	

Ana/Vo2 CARDIO INTERVALS
(Hvi's) mcw est. '13

	Date:	am or pm	Intervals:
	W.O.D.:	rps/rnds/lps	HrMx%
1			
2			
3			
4			
5			
6			
7			
8			
9			
10			
11			
12			
		A.L.O.I @:	

Ana/Vo2 CARDIO INTERVALS
(Hvi's) mcw est. '13

	Date:	am or pm	Intervals:
	W.O.D.:	rps/rnds/lps	HrMx%
1			
2			
3			
4			
5			
6			
7			
8			
9			
10			
11			
12			
		A.L.O.I @:	

Ana/Vo2 CARDIO INTERVALS
(Hvi's) mcw est. '13

	Date:	am or pm	Intervals:
	W.O.D.:	rps/rnds/lps	HrMx%
1			
2			
3			
4			
5			
6			
7			
8			
9			
10			
11			
12			
		A.L.O.I @:	

Ana/Vo2 CARDIO INTERVALS

(Hvi's) mcw est. '13

	Date:	am or pm	Intervals:
	W.O.D.:	rps/rnds/lps	HrMx%
1			
2			
3			
4			
5			
6			
7			
8			
9			
10			
11			
12			
		A.L.O.I @:	

Ana/Vo2 CARDIO INTERVALS

(Hvi's) mcw est. '13

	Date:	am or pm	Intervals:
	W.O.D.:	rps/rnds/lps	HrMx%
1			
2			
3			
4			
5			
6			
7			
8			
9			
10			
11			
12			
		A.L.O.I @:	

Ana/Vo2 CARDIO INTERVALS

(Hvi's) mcw est. '13

	Date:	am or pm	Intervals:
	W.O.D.:	rps/rnds/lps	HrMx%
1			
2			
3			
4			
5			
6			
7			
8			
9			
10			
11			
12			
		A.L.O.I @:	

Ana/Vo2 CARDIO INTERVALS

(Hvi's) mcw est. '13

	Date:	am or pm	Intervals:
	W.O.D.:	rps/rnds/lps	HrMx%
1			
2			
3			
4			
5			
6			
7			
8			
9			
10			
11			
12			
		A.L.O.I @:	

Ana/Vo2 CARDIO INTERVALS

(Hvi's) mcw est. '13

	Date:	am or pm	Intervals:
	W.O.D.:	rps/rnds/lps	HrMx%
1			
2			
3			
4			
5			
6			
7			
8			
9			
10			
11			
12			
		A.L.O.I @:	

Ana/Vo2 CARDIO INTERVALS

(Hvi's) mcw est. '13

	Date:	am or pm	Intervals:
	W.O.D.:	rps/rnds/lps	HrMx%
1			
2			
3			
4			
5			
6			
7			
8			
9			
10			
11			
12			
		A.L.O.I @:	

FITNESS EVOLUTION NOTES:

Track your Training Effort Intensity Level Zones, Calorie Expense, and Personal Benchmark Record Data

DATE:________ DATA:	DATE:________ DATA:
DATE:________ DATA:	DATE:________ DATA:
DATE:________ DATA:	DATE:________ DATA:
DATE:________ DATA:	DATE:________ DATA:
DATE:________ DATA:	DATE:________ DATA:
DATE:________ DATA:	DATE:________ DATA:
DATE:________ DATA:	DATE:________ DATA:

FITNESS EVOLUTION NOTES:	
Track your Training Effort Intensity Level Zones, Calorie Expense, and Personal Benchmark Record Data	
DATE:________ DATA:	DATE:________ DATA:
DATE:________ DATA:	DATE:________ DATA:
DATE:________ DATA:	DATE:________ DATA:
DATE:________ DATA:	DATE:________ DATA:
DATE:________ DATA:	DATE:________ DATA:
DATE:________ DATA:	DATE:________ DATA:
DATE:________ DATA:	DATE:________ DATA:

NOTES:

Notes:

6 Week Training Calendar

Month Year

SUNDAY	MONDAY	TUESDAY	WEDNESDAY	THURSDAY	FRIDAY	SATURDAY

Week 1

Date:	Date:	Date:	Date:	Date:	Date:	Date:
Mileage:	Mileage:	Mileage:	Mileage:	Mileage:	Mileage:	Mileage:

Week 2

Date:	Date:	Date:	Date:	Date:	Date:	Date:
Mileage:	Mileage:	Mileage:	Mileage:	Mileage:	Mileage:	Mileage:

Week 3

Date:	Date:	Date:	Date:	Date:	Date:	Date:
Mileage:	Mileage:	Mileage:	Mileage:	Mileage:	Mileage:	Mileage:

Week 4

Date:	Date:	Date:	Date:	Date:	Date:	Date:
Mileage:	Mileage:	Mileage:	Mileage:	Mileage:	Mileage:	Mileage:

Week 5

Date:	Date:	Date:	Date:	Date:	Date:	Date:
Mileage:	Mileage:	Mileage:	Mileage:	Mileage:	Mileage:	Mileage:

Week 6

Date:	Date:	Date:	Date:	Date:	Date:	Date:
Mileage:	Mileage:	Mileage:	Mileage:	Mileage:	Mileage:	Mileage:

Ana/Vo2 CARDIO INTERVALS
(Hvi's) mcw est. '13

	Date:	am or pm	Intervals:
	W.O.D.:	rps/rnds/lps	HrMx%
1			
2			
3			
4			
5			
6			
7			
8			
9			
10			
11			
12			
		A.L.O.I @:	

Ana/Vo2 CARDIO INTERVALS
(Hvi's) mcw est. '13

	Date:	am or pm	Intervals:
	W.O.D.:	rps/rnds/lps	HrMx%
1			
2			
3			
4			
5			
6			
7			
8			
9			
10			
11			
12			
		A.L.O.I @:	

Ana/Vo2 CARDIO INTERVALS
(Hvi's) mcw est. '13

	Date:	am or pm	Intervals:
	W.O.D.:	rps/rnds/lps	HrMx%
1			
2			
3			
4			
5			
6			
7			
8			
9			
10			
11			
12			
		A.L.O.I @:	

Ana/Vo2 CARDIO INTERVALS
(Hvi's) mcw est. '13

	Date:	am or pm	Intervals:
	W.O.D.:	rps/rnds/lps	HrMx%
1			
2			
3			
4			
5			
6			
7			
8			
9			
10			
11			
12			
		A.L.O.I @:	

Ana/Vo2 CARDIO INTERVALS
(Hvi's) mcw est. '13

	Date:	am or pm	Intervals:
	W.O.D.:	rps/rnds/lps	HrMx%
1			
2			
3			
4			
5			
6			
7			
8			
9			
10			
11			
12			
		A.L.O.I @:	

Ana/Vo2 CARDIO INTERVALS
(Hvi's) mcw est. '13

	Date:	am or pm	Intervals:
	W.O.D.:	rps/rnds/lps	HrMx%
1			
2			
3			
4			
5			
6			
7			
8			
9			
10			
11			
12			
		A.L.O.I @:	

Ana/Vo2 CARDIO INTERVALS
(Hvi's) mcw est. '13

	Date:	am or pm	Intervals:
	W.O.D.:	rps/rnds/lps	HrMx%
1			
2			
3			
4			
5			
6			
7			
8			
9			
10			
11			
12			
		A.L.O.I @:	

Ana/Vo2 CARDIO INTERVALS
(Hvi's) mcw est. '13

	Date:	am or pm	Intervals:
	W.O.D.:	rps/rnds/lps	HrMx%
1			
2			
3			
4			
5			
6			
7			
8			
9			
10			
11			
12			
		A.L.O.I @:	

Ana/Vo2 CARDIO INTERVALS
(Hvi's) mcw est. '13

	Date:	am or pm	Intervals:
	W.O.D.:	rps/rnds/lps	HrMx%
1			
2			
3			
4			
5			
6			
7			
8			
9			
10			
11			
12			
		A.L.O.I @:	

Ana/Vo2 CARDIO INTERVALS
(Hvi's) mcw est. '13

	Date:	am or pm	Intervals:
	W.O.D.:	rps/rnds/lps	HrMx%
1			
2			
3			
4			
5			
6			
7			
8			
9			
10			
11			
12			
		A.L.O.I @:	

Ana/Vo2 CARDIO INTERVALS
(Hvi's) mcw est. '13

	Date:	am or pm	Intervals:
	W.O.D.:	rps/rnds/lps	HrMx%
1			
2			
3			
4			
5			
6			
7			
8			
9			
10			
11			
12			
		A.L.O.I @:	

Ana/Vo2 CARDIO INTERVALS
(Hvi's) mcw est. '13

	Date:	am or pm	Intervals:
	W.O.D.:	rps/rnds/lps	HrMx%
1			
2			
3			
4			
5			
6			
7			
8			
9			
10			
11			
12			
		A.L.O.I @:	

Ana/Vo2 CARDIO INTERVALS
(Hvi's) mcw est. '13

	Date:	am or pm	Intervals:
	W.O.D.:	rps/rnds/lps	HrMx%
1			
2			
3			
4			
5			
6			
7			
8			
9			
10			
11			
12			
		A.L.O.I @:	

Ana/Vo2 CARDIO INTERVALS
(Hvi's) mcw est. '13

	Date:	am or pm	Intervals:
	W.O.D.:	rps/rnds/lps	HrMx%
1			
2			
3			
4			
5			
6			
7			
8			
9			
10			
11			
12			
		A.L.O.I @:	

Ana/Vo2 CARDIO INTERVALS
(Hvi's) mcw est. '13

	Date:	am or pm	Intervals:
	W.O.D.:	rps/rnds/lps	HrMx%
1			
2			
3			
4			
5			
6			
7			
8			
9			
10			
11			
12			
		A.L.O.I @:	

Ana/Vo2 CARDIO INTERVALS
(Hvi's) mcw est. '13

	Date:	am or pm	Intervals:
	W.O.D.:	rps/rnds/lps	HrMx%
1			
2			
3			
4			
5			
6			
7			
8			
9			
10			
11			
12			
		A.L.O.I @:	

Ana/Vo2 CARDIO INTERVALS
(Hvi's) mcw est. '13

	Date:	am or pm	Intervals:
	W.O.D.:	rps/rnds/lps	HrMx%
1			
2			
3			
4			
5			
6			
7			
8			
9			
10			
11			
12			
		A.L.O.I @:	

Ana/Vo2 CARDIO INTERVALS
(Hvi's) mcw est. '13

	Date:	am or pm	Intervals:
	W.O.D.:	rps/rnds/lps	HrMx%
1			
2			
3			
4			
5			
6			
7			
8			
9			
10			
11			
12			
		A.L.O.I @:	

Ana/Vo2 CARDIO INTERVALS

(Hvi's) mcw est. '13

	Date:	am or pm	Intervals:
	W.O.D.:	rps/rnds/lps	HrMx%
1			
2			
3			
4			
5			
6			
7			
8			
9			
10			
11			
12			
		A.L.O.I @:	

Ana/Vo2 CARDIO INTERVALS

(Hvi's) mcw est. '13

	Date:	am or pm	Intervals:
	W.O.D.:	rps/rnds/lps	HrMx%
1			
2			
3			
4			
5			
6			
7			
8			
9			
10			
11			
12			
		A.L.O.I @:	

Ana/Vo2 CARDIO INTERVALS

(Hvi's) mcw est. '13

	Date:	am or pm	Intervals:
	W.O.D.:	rps/rnds/lps	HrMx%
1			
2			
3			
4			
5			
6			
7			
8			
9			
10			
11			
12			
		A.L.O.I @:	

Ana/Vo2 CARDIO INTERVALS

(Hvi's) mcw est. '13

	Date:	am or pm	Intervals:
	W.O.D.:	rps/rnds/lps	HrMx%
1			
2			
3			
4			
5			
6			
7			
8			
9			
10			
11			
12			
		A.L.O.I @:	

Ana/Vo2 CARDIO INTERVALS

(Hvi's) mcw est. '13

	Date:	am or pm	Intervals:
	W.O.D.:	rps/rnds/lps	HrMx%
1			
2			
3			
4			
5			
6			
7			
8			
9			
10			
11			
12			
		A.L.O.I @:	

Ana/Vo2 CARDIO INTERVALS

(Hvi's) mcw est. '13

	Date:	am or pm	Intervals:
	W.O.D.:	rps/rnds/lps	HrMx%
1			
2			
3			
4			
5			
6			
7			
8			
9			
10			
11			
12			
		A.L.O.I @:	

Ana/Vo2 CARDIO INTERVALS
(Hvi's) mcw est. '13

	Date:	am or pm	Intervals:
	W.O.D.:	rps/rnds/lps	HrMx%
1			
2			
3			
4			
5			
6			
7			
8			
9			
10			
11			
12			
		A.L.O.I @:	

Ana/Vo2 CARDIO INTERVALS
(Hvi's) mcw est. '13

	Date:	am or pm	Intervals:
	W.O.D.:	rps/rnds/lps	HrMx%
1			
2			
3			
4			
5			
6			
7			
8			
9			
10			
11			
12			
		A.L.O.I @:	

Ana/Vo2 CARDIO INTERVALS
(Hvi's) mcw est. '13

	Date:	am or pm	Intervals:
	W.O.D.:	rps/rnds/lps	HrMx%
1			
2			
3			
4			
5			
6			
7			
8			
9			
10			
11			
12			
		A.L.O.I @:	

Ana/Vo2 CARDIO INTERVALS
(Hvi's) mcw est. '13

	Date:	am or pm	Intervals:
	W.O.D.:	rps/rnds/lps	HrMx%
1			
2			
3			
4			
5			
6			
7			
8			
9			
10			
11			
12			
		A.L.O.I @:	

Ana/Vo2 CARDIO INTERVALS
(Hvi's) mcw est. '13

	Date:	am or pm	Intervals:
	W.O.D.:	rps/rnds/lps	HrMx%
1			
2			
3			
4			
5			
6			
7			
8			
9			
10			
11			
12			
		A.L.O.I @:	

Ana/Vo2 CARDIO INTERVALS
(Hvi's) mcw est. '13

	Date:	am or pm	Intervals:
	W.O.D.:	rps/rnds/lps	HrMx%
1			
2			
3			
4			
5			
6			
7			
8			
9			
10			
11			
12			
		A.L.O.I @:	

FITNESS EVOLUTION NOTES:

Track your Training Effort Intensity Level Zones, Calorie Expense, and Personal Benchmark Record Data

DATE:__________ DATA:	DATE:__________ DATA:
DATE:__________ DATA:	DATE:__________ DATA:
DATE:__________ DATA:	DATE:__________ DATA:
DATE:__________ DATA:	DATE:__________ DATA:
DATE:__________ DATA:	DATE:__________ DATA:
DATE:__________ DATA:	DATE:__________ DATA:
DATE:__________ DATA:	DATE:__________ DATA:

FITNESS EVOLUTION NOTES:

Track your Training Effort Intensity Level Zones, Calorie Expense, and Personal Benchmark Record Data

DATE: DATA:	DATE: DATA:
DATE: DATA:	DATE: DATA:
DATE: DATA:	DATE: DATA:
DATE: DATA:	DATE: DATA:
DATE: DATA:	DATE: DATA:
DATE: DATA:	DATE: DATA:
DATE: DATA:	DATE: DATA:

NOTES:

NOTES:

6 Week Training Calendar

Month Year

SUNDAY	MONDAY	TUESDAY	WEDNESDAY	THURSDAY	FRIDAY	SATURDAY

Week 1

Date:	Date:	Date:	Date:	Date:	Date:	Date:
Mileage:	Mileage:	Mileage:	Mileage:	Mileage:	Mileage:	Mileage:

Week 2

Date:	Date:	Date:	Date:	Date:	Date:	Date:
Mileage:	Mileage:	Mileage:	Mileage:	Mileage:	Mileage:	Mileage:

Week 3

Date:	Date:	Date:	Date:	Date:	Date:	Date:
Mileage:	Mileage:	Mileage:	Mileage:	Mileage:	Mileage:	Mileage:

Week 4

Date:	Date:	Date:	Date:	Date:	Date:	Date:
Mileage:	Mileage:	Mileage:	Mileage:	Mileage:	Mileage:	Mileage:

Week 5

Date:	Date:	Date:	Date:	Date:	Date:	Date:
Mileage:	Mileage:	Mileage:	Mileage:	Mileage:	Mileage:	Mileage:

Week 6

Date:	Date:	Date:	Date:	Date:	Date:	Date:
Mileage:	Mileage:	Mileage:	Mileage:	Mileage:	Mileage:	Mileage:

Ana/Vo2 CARDIO INTERVALS
(Hvi's) mcw est. '13

	Date:	am or pm	Intervals:
	W.O.D.:	rps/rnds/lps	HrMx%
1			
2			
3			
4			
5			
6			
7			
8			
9			
10			
11			
12			
		A.L.O.I @:	

Ana/Vo2 CARDIO INTERVALS
(Hvi's) mcw est. '13

	Date:	am or pm	Intervals:
	W.O.D.:	rps/rnds/lps	HrMx%
1			
2			
3			
4			
5			
6			
7			
8			
9			
10			
11			
12			
		A.L.O.I @:	

Ana/Vo2 CARDIO INTERVALS
(Hvi's) mcw est. '13

	Date:	am or pm	Intervals:
	W.O.D.:	rps/rnds/lps	HrMx%
1			
2			
3			
4			
5			
6			
7			
8			
9			
10			
11			
12			
		A.L.O.I @:	

Ana/Vo2 CARDIO INTERVALS
(Hvi's) mcw est. '13

	Date:	am or pm	Intervals:
	W.O.D.:	rps/rnds/lps	HrMx%
1			
2			
3			
4			
5			
6			
7			
8			
9			
10			
11			
12			
		A.L.O.I @:	

Ana/Vo2 CARDIO INTERVALS
(Hvi's) mcw est. '13

	Date:	am or pm	Intervals:
	W.O.D.:	rps/rnds/lps	HrMx%
1			
2			
3			
4			
5			
6			
7			
8			
9			
10			
11			
12			
		A.L.O.I @:	

Ana/Vo2 CARDIO INTERVALS
(Hvi's) mcw est. '13

	Date:	am or pm	Intervals:
	W.O.D.:	rps/rnds/lps	HrMx%
1			
2			
3			
4			
5			
6			
7			
8			
9			
10			
11			
12			
		A.L.O.I @:	

Ana/Vo2 CARDIO INTERVALS
(Hvi's) mcw est. '13

	Date:	am or pm	Intervals:
	W.O.D.:	rps/rnds/lps	HrMx%
1			
2			
3			
4			
5			
6			
7			
8			
9			
10			
11			
12			
		A.L.O.I @:	

Ana/Vo2 CARDIO INTERVALS
(Hvi's) mcw est. '13

	Date:	am or pm	Intervals:
	W.O.D.:	rps/rnds/lps	HrMx%
1			
2			
3			
4			
5			
6			
7			
8			
9			
10			
11			
12			
		A.L.O.I @:	

Ana/Vo2 CARDIO INTERVALS
(Hvi's) mcw est. '13

	Date:	am or pm	Intervals:
	W.O.D.:	rps/rnds/lps	HrMx%
1			
2			
3			
4			
5			
6			
7			
8			
9			
10			
11			
12			
		A.L.O.I @:	

Ana/Vo2 CARDIO INTERVALS
(Hvi's) mcw est. '13

	Date:	am or pm	Intervals:
	W.O.D.:	rps/rnds/lps	HrMx%
1			
2			
3			
4			
5			
6			
7			
8			
9			
10			
11			
12			
		A.L.O.I @:	

Ana/Vo2 CARDIO INTERVALS
(Hvi's) mcw est. '13

	Date:	am or pm	Intervals:
	W.O.D.:	rps/rnds/lps	HrMx%
1			
2			
3			
4			
5			
6			
7			
8			
9			
10			
11			
12			
		A.L.O.I @:	

Ana/Vo2 CARDIO INTERVALS
(Hvi's) mcw est. '13

	Date:	am or pm	Intervals:
	W.O.D.:	rps/rnds/lps	HrMx%
1			
2			
3			
4			
5			
6			
7			
8			
9			
10			
11			
12			
		A.L.O.I @:	

Ana/Vo2 CARDIO INTERVALS
(Hvi's) mcw est. '13

	Date:	am or pm	Intervals:
	W.O.D.:	rps/rnds/lps	HrMx%
1			
2			
3			
4			
5			
6			
7			
8			
9			
10			
11			
12			
		A.L.O.I @:	

Ana/Vo2 CARDIO INTERVALS
(Hvi's) mcw est. '13

	Date:	am or pm	Intervals:
	W.O.D.:	rps/rnds/lps	HrMx%
1			
2			
3			
4			
5			
6			
7			
8			
9			
10			
11			
12			
		A.L.O.I @:	

Ana/Vo2 CARDIO INTERVALS
(Hvi's) mcw est. '13

	Date:	am or pm	Intervals:
	W.O.D.:	rps/rnds/lps	HrMx%
1			
2			
3			
4			
5			
6			
7			
8			
9			
10			
11			
12			
		A.L.O.I @:	

Ana/Vo2 CARDIO INTERVALS
(Hvi's) mcw est. '13

	Date:	am or pm	Intervals:
	W.O.D.:	rps/rnds/lps	HrMx%
1			
2			
3			
4			
5			
6			
7			
8			
9			
10			
11			
12			
		A.L.O.I @:	

Ana/Vo2 CARDIO INTERVALS
(Hvi's) mcw est. '13

	Date:	am or pm	Intervals:
	W.O.D.:	rps/rnds/lps	HrMx%
1			
2			
3			
4			
5			
6			
7			
8			
9			
10			
11			
12			
		A.L.O.I @:	

Ana/Vo2 CARDIO INTERVALS
(Hvi's) mcw est. '13

	Date:	am or pm	Intervals:
	W.O.D.:	rps/rnds/lps	HrMx%
1			
2			
3			
4			
5			
6			
7			
8			
9			
10			
11			
12			
		A.L.O.I @:	

Ana/Vo2 CARDIO INTERVALS
(Hvi's) mcw est. '13

	Date:	am or pm	Intervals:
	W.O.D.:	rps/rnds/lps	HrMx%
1			
2			
3			
4			
5			
6			
7			
8			
9			
10			
11			
12			
		A.L.O.I @:	

Ana/Vo2 CARDIO INTERVALS
(Hvi's) mcw est. '13

	Date:	am or pm	Intervals:
	W.O.D.:	rps/rnds/lps	HrMx%
1			
2			
3			
4			
5			
6			
7			
8			
9			
10			
11			
12			
		A.L.O.I @:	

Ana/Vo2 CARDIO INTERVALS
(Hvi's) mcw est. '13

	Date:	am or pm	Intervals:
	W.O.D.:	rps/rnds/lps	HrMx%
1			
2			
3			
4			
5			
6			
7			
8			
9			
10			
11			
12			
		A.L.O.I @:	

Ana/Vo2 CARDIO INTERVALS
(Hvi's) mcw est. '13

	Date:	am or pm	Intervals:
	W.O.D.:	rps/rnds/lps	HrMx%
1			
2			
3			
4			
5			
6			
7			
8			
9			
10			
11			
12			
		A.L.O.I @:	

Ana/Vo2 CARDIO INTERVALS
(Hvi's) mcw est. '13

	Date:	am or pm	Intervals:
	W.O.D.:	rps/rnds/lps	HrMx%
1			
2			
3			
4			
5			
6			
7			
8			
9			
10			
11			
12			
		A.L.O.I @:	

Ana/Vo2 CARDIO INTERVALS
(Hvi's) mcw est. '13

	Date:	am or pm	Intervals:
	W.O.D.:	rps/rnds/lps	HrMx%
1			
2			
3			
4			
5			
6			
7			
8			
9			
10			
11			
12			
		A.L.O.I @:	

Ana/Vo2 CARDIO INTERVALS
(Hvi's) mcw est. '13

	Date:	am or pm	Intervals:
	W.O.D.:	rps/rnds/lps	HrMx%
1			
2			
3			
4			
5			
6			
7			
8			
9			
10			
11			
12			
		A.L.O.I @:	

Ana/Vo2 CARDIO INTERVALS
(Hvi's) mcw est. '13

	Date:	am or pm	Intervals:
	W.O.D.:	rps/rnds/lps	HrMx%
1			
2			
3			
4			
5			
6			
7			
8			
9			
10			
11			
12			
		A.L.O.I @:	

Ana/Vo2 CARDIO INTERVALS
(Hvi's) mcw est. '13

	Date:	am or pm	Intervals:
	W.O.D.:	rps/rnds/lps	HrMx%
1			
2			
3			
4			
5			
6			
7			
8			
9			
10			
11			
12			
		A.L.O.I @:	

Ana/Vo2 CARDIO INTERVALS
(Hvi's) mcw est. '13

	Date:	am or pm	Intervals:
	W.O.D.:	rps/rnds/lps	HrMx%
1			
2			
3			
4			
5			
6			
7			
8			
9			
10			
11			
12			
		A.L.O.I @:	

Ana/Vo2 CARDIO INTERVALS
(Hvi's) mcw est. '13

	Date:	am or pm	Intervals:
	W.O.D.:	rps/rnds/lps	HrMx%
1			
2			
3			
4			
5			
6			
7			
8			
9			
10			
11			
12			
		A.L.O.I @:	

Ana/Vo2 CARDIO INTERVALS
(Hvi's) mcw est. '13

	Date:	am or pm	Intervals:
	W.O.D.:	rps/rnds/lps	HrMx%
1			
2			
3			
4			
5			
6			
7			
8			
9			
10			
11			
12			
		A.L.O.I @:	

FITNESS EVOLUTION NOTES:

Track your Training Effort Intensity Level Zones, Calorie Expense, and Personal Benchmark Record Data

DATE:___________ DATA:	DATE:___________ DATA:
DATE:___________ DATA:	DATE:___________ DATA:
DATE:___________ DATA:	DATE:___________ DATA:
DATE:___________ DATA:	DATE:___________ DATA:
DATE:___________ DATA:	DATE:___________ DATA:
DATE:___________ DATA:	DATE:___________ DATA:
DATE:___________ DATA:	DATE:___________ DATA:

FITNESS EVOLUTION NOTES:

Track your Training Effort Intensity Level Zones, Calorie Expense, and Personal Benchmark Record Data

DATE:__________ DATA:	DATE:__________ DATA:
DATE:__________ DATA:	DATE:__________ DATA:
DATE:__________ DATA:	DATE:__________ DATA:
DATE:__________ DATA:	DATE:__________ DATA:
DATE:__________ DATA:	DATE:__________ DATA:
DATE:__________ DATA:	DATE:__________ DATA:
DATE:__________ DATA:	DATE:__________ DATA:

NOTES:

NOTES:

6 Week Training Calendar

Month Year

SUNDAY	MONDAY	TUESDAY	WEDNESDAY	THURSDAY	FRIDAY	SATURDAY

Week 1

Date:	Date:	Date:	Date:	Date:	Date:	Date:
Mileage:	Mileage:	Mileage:	Mileage:	Mileage:	Mileage:	Mileage:

Week 2

Date:	Date:	Date:	Date:	Date:	Date:	Date:
Mileage:	Mileage:	Mileage:	Mileage:	Mileage:	Mileage:	Mileage:

Week 3

Date:	Date:	Date:	Date:	Date:	Date:	Date:
Mileage:	Mileage:	Mileage:	Mileage:	Mileage:	Mileage:	Mileage:

Week 4

Date:	Date:	Date:	Date:	Date:	Date:	Date:
Mileage:	Mileage:	Mileage:	Mileage:	Mileage:	Mileage:	Mileage:

Week 5

Date:	Date:	Date:	Date:	Date:	Date:	Date:
Mileage:	Mileage:	Mileage:	Mileage:	Mileage:	Mileage:	Mileage:

Week 6

Date:	Date:	Date:	Date:	Date:	Date:	Date:
Mileage:	Mileage:	Mileage:	Mileage:	Mileage:	Mileage:	Mileage:

Ana/Vo2 CARDIO INTERVALS
(Hvi's) mcw est. '13

	Date:	am or pm	Intervals:
	W.O.D.:	rps/rnds/lps	HrMx%
1			
2			
3			
4			
5			
6			
7			
8			
9			
10			
11			
12			
		A.L.O.I @:	

Ana/Vo2 CARDIO INTERVALS
(Hvi's) mcw est. '13

	Date:	am or pm	Intervals:
	W.O.D.:	rps/rnds/lps	HrMx%
1			
2			
3			
4			
5			
6			
7			
8			
9			
10			
11			
12			
		A.L.O.I @:	

Ana/Vo2 CARDIO INTERVALS
(Hvi's) mcw est. '13

	Date:	am or pm	Intervals:
	W.O.D.:	rps/rnds/lps	HrMx%
1			
2			
3			
4			
5			
6			
7			
8			
9			
10			
11			
12			
		A.L.O.I @:	

Ana/Vo2 CARDIO INTERVALS
(Hvi's) mcw est. '13

	Date:	am or pm	Intervals:
	W.O.D.:	rps/rnds/lps	HrMx%
1			
2			
3			
4			
5			
6			
7			
8			
9			
10			
11			
12			
		A.L.O.I @:	

Ana/Vo2 CARDIO INTERVALS
(Hvi's) mcw est. '13

	Date:	am or pm	Intervals:
	W.O.D.:	rps/rnds/lps	HrMx%
1			
2			
3			
4			
5			
6			
7			
8			
9			
10			
11			
12			
		A.L.O.I @:	

Ana/Vo2 CARDIO INTERVALS
(Hvi's) mcw est. '13

	Date:	am or pm	Intervals:
	W.O.D.:	rps/rnds/lps	HrMx%
1			
2			
3			
4			
5			
6			
7			
8			
9			
10			
11			
12			
		A.L.O.I @:	

Ana/Vo2 CARDIO INTERVALS

(Hvi's) mcw est. '13

	Date:	am or pm	Intervals:
	W.O.D.:	rps/rnds/lps	HrMx%
1			
2			
3			
4			
5			
6			
7			
8			
9			
10			
11			
12			
		A.L.O.I @:	

Ana/Vo2 CARDIO INTERVALS

(Hvi's) mcw est. '13

	Date:	am or pm	Intervals:
	W.O.D.:	rps/rnds/lps	HrMx%
1			
2			
3			
4			
5			
6			
7			
8			
9			
10			
11			
12			
		A.L.O.I @:	

Ana/Vo2 CARDIO INTERVALS

(Hvi's) mcw est. '13

	Date:	am or pm	Intervals:
	W.O.D.:	rps/rnds/lps	HrMx%
1			
2			
3			
4			
5			
6			
7			
8			
9			
10			
11			
12			
		A.L.O.I @:	

Ana/Vo2 CARDIO INTERVALS

(Hvi's) mcw est. '13

	Date:	am or pm	Intervals:
	W.O.D.:	rps/rnds/lps	HrMx%
1			
2			
3			
4			
5			
6			
7			
8			
9			
10			
11			
12			
		A.L.O.I @:	

Ana/Vo2 CARDIO INTERVALS

(Hvi's) mcw est. '13

	Date:	am or pm	Intervals:
	W.O.D.:	rps/rnds/lps	HrMx%
1			
2			
3			
4			
5			
6			
7			
8			
9			
10			
11			
12			
		A.L.O.I @:	

Ana/Vo2 CARDIO INTERVALS

(Hvi's) mcw est. '13

	Date:	am or pm	Intervals:
	W.O.D.:	rps/rnds/lps	HrMx%
1			
2			
3			
4			
5			
6			
7			
8			
9			
10			
11			
12			
		A.L.O.I @:	

Ana/Vo2 CARDIO INTERVALS
(Hvi's) mcw est. '13

	Date:	am or pm	Intervals:
	W.O.D.:	rps/rnds/lps	HrMx%
1			
2			
3			
4			
5			
6			
7			
8			
9			
10			
11			
12			
		A.L.O.I @:	

Ana/Vo2 CARDIO INTERVALS
(Hvi's) mcw est. '13

	Date:	am or pm	Intervals:
	W.O.D.:	rps/rnds/lps	HrMx%
1			
2			
3			
4			
5			
6			
7			
8			
9			
10			
11			
12			
		A.L.O.I @:	

Ana/Vo2 CARDIO INTERVALS
(Hvi's) mcw est. '13

	Date:	am or pm	Intervals:
	W.O.D.:	rps/rnds/lps	HrMx%
1			
2			
3			
4			
5			
6			
7			
8			
9			
10			
11			
12			
		A.L.O.I @:	

Ana/Vo2 CARDIO INTERVALS
(Hvi's) mcw est. '13

	Date:	am or pm	Intervals:
	W.O.D.:	rps/rnds/lps	HrMx%
1			
2			
3			
4			
5			
6			
7			
8			
9			
10			
11			
12			
		A.L.O.I @:	

Ana/Vo2 CARDIO INTERVALS
(Hvi's) mcw est. '13

	Date:	am or pm	Intervals:
	W.O.D.:	rps/rnds/lps	HrMx%
1			
2			
3			
4			
5			
6			
7			
8			
9			
10			
11			
12			
		A.L.O.I @:	

Ana/Vo2 CARDIO INTERVALS
(Hvi's) mcw est. '13

	Date:	am or pm	Intervals:
	W.O.D.:	rps/rnds/lps	HrMx%
1			
2			
3			
4			
5			
6			
7			
8			
9			
10			
11			
12			
		A.L.O.I @:	

Ana/Vo2 CARDIO INTERVALS
(Hvi's) mcw est. '13

	Date:	am or pm	Intervals:
	W.O.D.:	rps/rnds/lps	HrMx%
1			
2			
3			
4			
5			
6			
7			
8			
9			
10			
11			
12			
		A.L.O.I @:	

Ana/Vo2 CARDIO INTERVALS
(Hvi's) mcw est. '13

	Date:	am or pm	Intervals:
	W.O.D.:	rps/rnds/lps	HrMx%
1			
2			
3			
4			
5			
6			
7			
8			
9			
10			
11			
12			
		A.L.O.I @:	

Ana/Vo2 CARDIO INTERVALS
(Hvi's) mcw est. '13

	Date:	am or pm	Intervals:
	W.O.D.:	rps/rnds/lps	HrMx%
1			
2			
3			
4			
5			
6			
7			
8			
9			
10			
11			
12			
		A.L.O.I @:	

Ana/Vo2 CARDIO INTERVALS
(Hvi's) mcw est. '13

	Date:	am or pm	Intervals:
	W.O.D.:	rps/rnds/lps	HrMx%
1			
2			
3			
4			
5			
6			
7			
8			
9			
10			
11			
12			
		A.L.O.I @:	

Ana/Vo2 CARDIO INTERVALS
(Hvi's) mcw est. '13

	Date:	am or pm	Intervals:
	W.O.D.:	rps/rnds/lps	HrMx%
1			
2			
3			
4			
5			
6			
7			
8			
9			
10			
11			
12			
		A.L.O.I @:	

Ana/Vo2 CARDIO INTERVALS
(Hvi's) mcw est. '13

	Date:	am or pm	Intervals:
	W.O.D.:	rps/rnds/lps	HrMx%
1			
2			
3			
4			
5			
6			
7			
8			
9			
10			
11			
12			
		A.L.O.I @:	

Ana/Vo2 CARDIO INTERVALS
(Hvi's) mcw est. '13

	Date:	am or pm	Intervals:
	W.O.D.:	rps/rnds/lps	HrMx%
1			
2			
3			
4			
5			
6			
7			
8			
9			
10			
11			
12			
		A.L.O.I @:	

Ana/Vo2 CARDIO INTERVALS
(Hvi's) mcw est. '13

	Date:	am or pm	Intervals:
	W.O.D.:	rps/rnds/lps	HrMx%
1			
2			
3			
4			
5			
6			
7			
8			
9			
10			
11			
12			
		A.L.O.I @:	

Ana/Vo2 CARDIO INTERVALS
(Hvi's) mcw est. '13

	Date:	am or pm	Intervals:
	W.O.D.:	rps/rnds/lps	HrMx%
1			
2			
3			
4			
5			
6			
7			
8			
9			
10			
11			
12			
		A.L.O.I @:	

Ana/Vo2 CARDIO INTERVALS
(Hvi's) mcw est. '13

	Date:	am or pm	Intervals:
	W.O.D.:	rps/rnds/lps	HrMx%
1			
2			
3			
4			
5			
6			
7			
8			
9			
10			
11			
12			
		A.L.O.I @:	

Ana/Vo2 CARDIO INTERVALS
(Hvi's) mcw est. '13

	Date:	am or pm	Intervals:
	W.O.D.:	rps/rnds/lps	HrMx%
1			
2			
3			
4			
5			
6			
7			
8			
9			
10			
11			
12			
		A.L.O.I @:	

Ana/Vo2 CARDIO INTERVALS
(Hvi's) mcw est. '13

	Date:	am or pm	Intervals:
	W.O.D.:	rps/rnds/lps	HrMx%
1			
2			
3			
4			
5			
6			
7			
8			
9			
10			
11			
12			
		A.L.O.I @:	

FITNESS EVOLUTION NOTES:

Track your Training Effort Intensity Level Zones, Calorie Expense, and Personal Benchmark Record Data

DATE:________ DATA:	DATE:________ DATA:
DATE:________ DATA:	DATE:________ DATA:
DATE:________ DATA:	DATE:________ DATA:
DATE:________ DATA:	DATE:________ DATA:
DATE:________ DATA:	DATE:________ DATA:
DATE:________ DATA:	DATE:________ DATA:
DATE:________ DATA:	DATE:________ DATA:

FITNESS EVOLUTION NOTES:

Track your Training Effort Intensity Level Zones, Calorie Expense, and Personal Benchmark Record Data

DATE:_______ DATA:	DATE:_______ DATA:
DATE:_______ DATA:	DATE:_______ DATA:
DATE:_______ DATA:	DATE:_______ DATA:
DATE:_______ DATA:	DATE:_______ DATA:
DATE:_______ DATA:	DATE:_______ DATA:
DATE:_______ DATA:	DATE:_______ DATA:
DATE:_______ DATA:	DATE:_______ DATA:

NOTES:

NOTES:

6 Week Training Calendar

Month Year

SUNDAY	MONDAY	TUESDAY	WEDNESDAY	THURSDAY	FRIDAY	SATURDAY

Week 1

Date:	Date:	Date:	Date:	Date:	Date:	Date:
Mileage:	Mileage:	Mileage:	Mileage:	Mileage:	Mileage:	Mileage:

Week 2

Date:	Date:	Date:	Date:	Date:	Date:	Date:
Mileage:	Mileage:	Mileage:	Mileage:	Mileage:	Mileage:	Mileage:

Week 3

Date:	Date:	Date:	Date:	Date:	Date:	Date:
Mileage:	Mileage:	Mileage:	Mileage:	Mileage:	Mileage:	Mileage:

Week 4

Date:	Date:	Date:	Date:	Date:	Date:	Date:
Mileage:	Mileage:	Mileage:	Mileage:	Mileage:	Mileage:	Mileage:

Week 5

Date:	Date:	Date:	Date:	Date:	Date:	Date:
Mileage:	Mileage:	Mileage:	Mileage:	Mileage:	Mileage:	Mileage:

Week 6

Date:	Date:	Date:	Date:	Date:	Date:	Date:
Mileage:	Mileage:	Mileage:	Mileage:	Mileage:	Mileage:	Mileage:

Ana/Vo2 CARDIO INTERVALS
(Hvi's) mcw est. '13

	Date:	am or pm	Intervals:
	W.O.D.:	rps/rnds/lps	HrMx%
1			
2			
3			
4			
5			
6			
7			
8			
9			
10			
11			
12			
		A.L.O.I @:	

Ana/Vo2 CARDIO INTERVALS
(Hvi's) mcw est. '13

	Date:	am or pm	Intervals:
	W.O.D.:	rps/rnds/lps	HrMx%
1			
2			
3			
4			
5			
6			
7			
8			
9			
10			
11			
12			
		A.L.O.I @:	

Ana/Vo2 CARDIO INTERVALS
(Hvi's) mcw est. '13

	Date:	am or pm	Intervals:
	W.O.D.:	rps/rnds/lps	HrMx%
1			
2			
3			
4			
5			
6			
7			
8			
9			
10			
11			
12			
		A.L.O.I @:	

Ana/Vo2 CARDIO INTERVALS
(Hvi's) mcw est. '13

	Date:	am or pm	Intervals:
	W.O.D.:	rps/rnds/lps	HrMx%
1			
2			
3			
4			
5			
6			
7			
8			
9			
10			
11			
12			
		A.L.O.I @:	

Ana/Vo2 CARDIO INTERVALS
(Hvi's) mcw est. '13

	Date:	am or pm	Intervals:
	W.O.D.:	rps/rnds/lps	HrMx%
1			
2			
3			
4			
5			
6			
7			
8			
9			
10			
11			
12			
		A.L.O.I @:	

Ana/Vo2 CARDIO INTERVALS
(Hvi's) mcw est. '13

	Date:	am or pm	Intervals:
	W.O.D.:	rps/rnds/lps	HrMx%
1			
2			
3			
4			
5			
6			
7			
8			
9			
10			
11			
12			
		A.L.O.I @:	

Ana/Vo2 CARDIO INTERVALS
(Hvi's) mcw est. '13

	Date:	am or pm	Intervals:
	W.O.D.:	rps/rnds/lps	HrMx%
1			
2			
3			
4			
5			
6			
7			
8			
9			
10			
11			
12			
		A.L.O.I @:	

Ana/Vo2 CARDIO INTERVALS
(Hvi's) mcw est. '13

	Date:	am or pm	Intervals:
	W.O.D.:	rps/rnds/lps	HrMx%
1			
2			
3			
4			
5			
6			
7			
8			
9			
10			
11			
12			
		A.L.O.I @:	

Ana/Vo2 CARDIO INTERVALS
(Hvi's) mcw est. '13

	Date:	am or pm	Intervals:
	W.O.D.:	rps/rnds/lps	HrMx%
1			
2			
3			
4			
5			
6			
7			
8			
9			
10			
11			
12			
		A.L.O.I @:	

Ana/Vo2 CARDIO INTERVALS
(Hvi's) mcw est. '13

	Date:	am or pm	Intervals:
	W.O.D.:	rps/rnds/lps	HrMx%
1			
2			
3			
4			
5			
6			
7			
8			
9			
10			
11			
12			
		A.L.O.I @:	

Ana/Vo2 CARDIO INTERVALS
(Hvi's) mcw est. '13

	Date:	am or pm	Intervals:
	W.O.D.:	rps/rnds/lps	HrMx%
1			
2			
3			
4			
5			
6			
7			
8			
9			
10			
11			
12			
		A.L.O.I @:	

Ana/Vo2 CARDIO INTERVALS
(Hvi's) mcw est. '13

	Date:	am or pm	Intervals:
	W.O.D.:	rps/rnds/lps	HrMx%
1			
2			
3			
4			
5			
6			
7			
8			
9			
10			
11			
12			
		A.L.O.I @:	

Ana/Vo2 CARDIO INTERVALS
(Hvi's) mcw est. '13

	Date:	am or pm	Intervals:
	W.O.D.:	rps/rnds/lps	HrMx%
1			
2			
3			
4			
5			
6			
7			
8			
9			
10			
11			
12			
		A.L.O.I @:	

Ana/Vo2 CARDIO INTERVALS
(Hvi's) mcw est. '13

	Date:	am or pm	Intervals:
	W.O.D.:	rps/rnds/lps	HrMx%
1			
2			
3			
4			
5			
6			
7			
8			
9			
10			
11			
12			
		A.L.O.I @:	

Ana/Vo2 CARDIO INTERVALS
(Hvi's) mcw est. '13

	Date:	am or pm	Intervals:
	W.O.D.:	rps/rnds/lps	HrMx%
1			
2			
3			
4			
5			
6			
7			
8			
9			
10			
11			
12			
		A.L.O.I @:	

Ana/Vo2 CARDIO INTERVALS
(Hvi's) mcw est. '13

	Date:	am or pm	Intervals:
	W.O.D.:	rps/rnds/lps	HrMx%
1			
2			
3			
4			
5			
6			
7			
8			
9			
10			
11			
12			
		A.L.O.I @:	

Ana/Vo2 CARDIO INTERVALS
(Hvi's) mcw est. '13

	Date:	am or pm	Intervals:
	W.O.D.:	rps/rnds/lps	HrMx%
1			
2			
3			
4			
5			
6			
7			
8			
9			
10			
11			
12			
		A.L.O.I @:	

Ana/Vo2 CARDIO INTERVALS
(Hvi's) mcw est. '13

	Date:	am or pm	Intervals:
	W.O.D.:	rps/rnds/lps	HrMx%
1			
2			
3			
4			
5			
6			
7			
8			
9			
10			
11			
12			
		A.L.O.I @:	

Ana/Vo2 CARDIO INTERVALS

(Hvi's) mcw est. '13

	Date:	am or pm	Intervals:
	W.O.D.:	rps/rnds/lps	HrMx%
1			
2			
3			
4			
5			
6			
7			
8			
9			
10			
11			
12			
		A.L.O.I @:	

Ana/Vo2 CARDIO INTERVALS

(Hvi's) mcw est. '13

	Date:	am or pm	Intervals:
	W.O.D.:	rps/rnds/lps	HrMx%
1			
2			
3			
4			
5			
6			
7			
8			
9			
10			
11			
12			
		A.L.O.I @:	

Ana/Vo2 CARDIO INTERVALS

(Hvi's) mcw est. '13

	Date:	am or pm	Intervals:
	W.O.D.:	rps/rnds/lps	HrMx%
1			
2			
3			
4			
5			
6			
7			
8			
9			
10			
11			
12			
		A.L.O.I @:	

Ana/Vo2 CARDIO INTERVALS

(Hvi's) mcw est. '13

	Date:	am or pm	Intervals:
	W.O.D.:	rps/rnds/lps	HrMx%
1			
2			
3			
4			
5			
6			
7			
8			
9			
10			
11			
12			
		A.L.O.I @:	

Ana/Vo2 CARDIO INTERVALS

(Hvi's) mcw est. '13

	Date:	am or pm	Intervals:
	W.O.D.:	rps/rnds/lps	HrMx%
1			
2			
3			
4			
5			
6			
7			
8			
9			
10			
11			
12			
		A.L.O.I @:	

Ana/Vo2 CARDIO INTERVALS

(Hvi's) mcw est. '13

	Date:	am or pm	Intervals:
	W.O.D.:	rps/rnds/lps	HrMx%
1			
2			
3			
4			
5			
6			
7			
8			
9			
10			
11			
12			
		A.L.O.I @:	

Ana/Vo2 CARDIO INTERVALS

(Hvi's) mcw est. '13

	Date:	am or pm	Intervals:
	W.O.D.:	rps/rnds/lps	HrMx%
1			
2			
3			
4			
5			
6			
7			
8			
9			
10			
11			
12			
		A.L.O.I @:	

Ana/Vo2 CARDIO INTERVALS

(Hvi's) mcw est. '13

	Date:	am or pm	Intervals:
	W.O.D.:	rps/rnds/lps	HrMx%
1			
2			
3			
4			
5			
6			
7			
8			
9			
10			
11			
12			
		A.L.O.I @:	

Ana/Vo2 CARDIO INTERVALS

(Hvi's) mcw est. '13

	Date:	am or pm	Intervals:
	W.O.D.:	rps/rnds/lps	HrMx%
1			
2			
3			
4			
5			
6			
7			
8			
9			
10			
11			
12			
		A.L.O.I @:	

Ana/Vo2 CARDIO INTERVALS

(Hvi's) mcw est. '13

	Date:	am or pm	Intervals:
	W.O.D.:	rps/rnds/lps	HrMx%
1			
2			
3			
4			
5			
6			
7			
8			
9			
10			
11			
12			
		A.L.O.I @:	

Ana/Vo2 CARDIO INTERVALS

(Hvi's) mcw est. '13

	Date:	am or pm	Intervals:
	W.O.D.:	rps/rnds/lps	HrMx%
1			
2			
3			
4			
5			
6			
7			
8			
9			
10			
11			
12			
		A.L.O.I @:	

Ana/Vo2 CARDIO INTERVALS

(Hvi's) mcw est. '13

	Date:	am or pm	Intervals:
	W.O.D.:	rps/rnds/lps	HrMx%
1			
2			
3			
4			
5			
6			
7			
8			
9			
10			
11			
12			
		A.L.O.I @:	

FITNESS EVOLUTION NOTES:

Track your Training Effort Intensity Level Zones, Calorie Expense, and Personal Benchmark Record Data

DATE:________ DATA:	DATE:________ DATA:
DATE:________ DATA:	DATE:________ DATA:
DATE:________ DATA:	DATE:________ DATA:
DATE:________ DATA:	DATE:________ DATA:
DATE:________ DATA:	DATE:________ DATA:
DATE:________ DATA:	DATE:________ DATA:
DATE:________ DATA:	DATE:________ DATA:

FITNESS EVOLUTION NOTES:

Track your Training Effort Intensity Level Zones, Calorie Expense, and Personal Benchmark Record Data

DATE:_________ DATA:	DATE:_________ DATA:
DATE:_________ DATA:	DATE:_________ DATA:
DATE:_________ DATA:	DATE:_________ DATA:
DATE:_________ DATA:	DATE:_________ DATA:
DATE:_________ DATA:	DATE:_________ DATA:
DATE:_________ DATA:	DATE:_________ DATA:
DATE:_________ DATA:	DATE:_________ DATA:

NOTES:

NOTES:

6 Week Training Calendar

Month Year

SUNDAY	MONDAY	TUESDAY	WEDNESDAY	THURSDAY	FRIDAY	SATURDAY
Week 1						
Date:	Date:	Date:	Date:	Date:	Date:	Date:
Mileage:	Mileage:	Mileage:	Mileage:	Mileage:	Mileage:	Mileage:
Week 2						
Date:	Date:	Date:	Date:	Date:	Date:	Date:
Mileage:	Mileage:	Mileage:	Mileage:	Mileage:	Mileage:	Mileage:
Week 3						
Date:	Date:	Date:	Date:	Date:	Date:	Date:
Mileage:	Mileage:	Mileage:	Mileage:	Mileage:	Mileage:	Mileage:
Week 4						
Date:	Date:	Date:	Date:	Date:	Date:	Date:
Mileage:	Mileage:	Mileage:	Mileage:	Mileage:	Mileage:	Mileage:
Week 5						
Date:	Date:	Date:	Date:	Date:	Date:	Date:
Mileage:	Mileage:	Mileage:	Mileage:	Mileage:	Mileage:	Mileage:
Week 6						
Date:	Date:	Date:	Date:	Date:	Date:	Date:
Mileage:	Mileage:	Mileage:	Mileage:	Mileage:	Mileage:	Mileage:

Ana/Vo2 CARDIO INTERVALS
(Hvi's) mcw est. '13

	Date:	am or pm	Intervals:
	W.O.D.:	rps/rnds/lps	HrMx%
1			
2			
3			
4			
5			
6			
7			
8			
9			
10			
11			
12			
		A.L.O.I @:	

Ana/Vo2 CARDIO INTERVALS
(Hvi's) mcw est. '13

	Date:	am or pm	Intervals:
	W.O.D.:	rps/rnds/lps	HrMx%
1			
2			
3			
4			
5			
6			
7			
8			
9			
10			
11			
12			
		A.L.O.I @:	

Ana/Vo2 CARDIO INTERVALS
(Hvi's) mcw est. '13

	Date:	am or pm	Intervals:
	W.O.D.:	rps/rnds/lps	HrMx%
1			
2			
3			
4			
5			
6			
7			
8			
9			
10			
11			
12			
		A.L.O.I @:	

Ana/Vo2 CARDIO INTERVALS
(Hvi's) mcw est. '13

	Date:	am or pm	Intervals:
	W.O.D.:	rps/rnds/lps	HrMx%
1			
2			
3			
4			
5			
6			
7			
8			
9			
10			
11			
12			
		A.L.O.I @:	

Ana/Vo2 CARDIO INTERVALS
(Hvi's) mcw est. '13

	Date:	am or pm	Intervals:
	W.O.D.:	rps/rnds/lps	HrMx%
1			
2			
3			
4			
5			
6			
7			
8			
9			
10			
11			
12			
		A.L.O.I @:	

Ana/Vo2 CARDIO INTERVALS
(Hvi's) mcw est. '13

	Date:	am or pm	Intervals:
	W.O.D.:	rps/rnds/lps	HrMx%
1			
2			
3			
4			
5			
6			
7			
8			
9			
10			
11			
12			
		A.L.O.I @:	

Ana/Vo2 CARDIO INTERVALS

(Hvi's) mcw est. '13

	Date:	am or pm	Intervals:
	W.O.D.:	rps/rnds/lps	HrMx%
1			
2			
3			
4			
5			
6			
7			
8			
9			
10			
11			
12			
		A.L.O.I @:	

Ana/Vo2 CARDIO INTERVALS

(Hvi's) mcw est. '13

	Date:	am or pm	Intervals:
	W.O.D.:	rps/rnds/lps	HrMx%
1			
2			
3			
4			
5			
6			
7			
8			
9			
10			
11			
12			
		A.L.O.I @:	

Ana/Vo2 CARDIO INTERVALS

(Hvi's) mcw est. '13

	Date:	am or pm	Intervals:
	W.O.D.:	rps/rnds/lps	HrMx%
1			
2			
3			
4			
5			
6			
7			
8			
9			
10			
11			
12			
		A.L.O.I @:	

Ana/Vo2 CARDIO INTERVALS

(Hvi's) mcw est. '13

	Date:	am or pm	Intervals:
	W.O.D.:	rps/rnds/lps	HrMx%
1			
2			
3			
4			
5			
6			
7			
8			
9			
10			
11			
12			
		A.L.O.I @:	

Ana/Vo2 CARDIO INTERVALS

(Hvi's) mcw est. '13

	Date:	am or pm	Intervals:
	W.O.D.:	rps/rnds/lps	HrMx%
1			
2			
3			
4			
5			
6			
7			
8			
9			
10			
11			
12			
		A.L.O.I @:	

Ana/Vo2 CARDIO INTERVALS

(Hvi's) mcw est. '13

	Date:	am or pm	Intervals:
	W.O.D.:	rps/rnds/lps	HrMx%
1			
2			
3			
4			
5			
6			
7			
8			
9			
10			
11			
12			
		A.L.O.I @:	

Ana/Vo2 CARDIO INTERVALS
(Hvi's) mcw est. '13

	Date:	am or pm	Intervals:
	W.O.D.:	rps/rnds/lps	HrMx%
1			
2			
3			
4			
5			
6			
7			
8			
9			
10			
11			
12			
		A.L.O.I @:	

Ana/Vo2 CARDIO INTERVALS
(Hvi's) mcw est. '13

	Date:	am or pm	Intervals:
	W.O.D.:	rps/rnds/lps	HrMx%
1			
2			
3			
4			
5			
6			
7			
8			
9			
10			
11			
12			
		A.L.O.I @:	

Ana/Vo2 CARDIO INTERVALS
(Hvi's) mcw est. '13

	Date:	am or pm	Intervals:
	W.O.D.:	rps/rnds/lps	HrMx%
1			
2			
3			
4			
5			
6			
7			
8			
9			
10			
11			
12			
		A.L.O.I @:	

Ana/Vo2 CARDIO INTERVALS
(Hvi's) mcw est. '13

	Date:	am or pm	Intervals:
	W.O.D.:	rps/rnds/lps	HrMx%
1			
2			
3			
4			
5			
6			
7			
8			
9			
10			
11			
12			
		A.L.O.I @:	

Ana/Vo2 CARDIO INTERVALS
(Hvi's) mcw est. '13

	Date:	am or pm	Intervals:
	W.O.D.:	rps/rnds/lps	HrMx%
1			
2			
3			
4			
5			
6			
7			
8			
9			
10			
11			
12			
		A.L.O.I @:	

Ana/Vo2 CARDIO INTERVALS
(Hvi's) mcw est. '13

	Date:	am or pm	Intervals:
	W.O.D.:	rps/rnds/lps	HrMx%
1			
2			
3			
4			
5			
6			
7			
8			
9			
10			
11			
12			
		A.L.O.I @:	

Ana/Vo2 CARDIO INTERVALS
(Hvi's) mcw est. '13

	Date:	am or pm	Intervals:
	W.O.D.:	rps/rnds/lps	HrMx%
1			
2			
3			
4			
5			
6			
7			
8			
9			
10			
11			
12			
		A.L.O.I @:	

Ana/Vo2 CARDIO INTERVALS
(Hvi's) mcw est. '13

	Date:	am or pm	Intervals:
	W.O.D.:	rps/rnds/lps	HrMx%
1			
2			
3			
4			
5			
6			
7			
8			
9			
10			
11			
12			
		A.L.O.I @:	

Ana/Vo2 CARDIO INTERVALS
(Hvi's) mcw est. '13

	Date:	am or pm	Intervals:
	W.O.D.:	rps/rnds/lps	HrMx%
1			
2			
3			
4			
5			
6			
7			
8			
9			
10			
11			
12			
		A.L.O.I @:	

Ana/Vo2 CARDIO INTERVALS
(Hvi's) mcw est. '13

	Date:	am or pm	Intervals:
	W.O.D.:	rps/rnds/lps	HrMx%
1			
2			
3			
4			
5			
6			
7			
8			
9			
10			
11			
12			
		A.L.O.I @:	

Ana/Vo2 CARDIO INTERVALS
(Hvi's) mcw est. '13

	Date:	am or pm	Intervals:
	W.O.D.:	rps/rnds/lps	HrMx%
1			
2			
3			
4			
5			
6			
7			
8			
9			
10			
11			
12			
		A.L.O.I @:	

Ana/Vo2 CARDIO INTERVALS
(Hvi's) mcw est. '13

	Date:	am or pm	Intervals:
	W.O.D.:	rps/rnds/lps	HrMx%
1			
2			
3			
4			
5			
6			
7			
8			
9			
10			
11			
12			
		A.L.O.I @:	

Ana/Vo2 CARDIO INTERVALS
(Hvi's) mcw est. '13

	Date:	am or pm	Intervals:
	W.O.D.:	rps/rnds/lps	HrMx%
1			
2			
3			
4			
5			
6			
7			
8			
9			
10			
11			
12			
		A.L.O.I @:	

Ana/Vo2 CARDIO INTERVALS
(Hvi's) mcw est. '13

	Date:	am or pm	Intervals:
	W.O.D.:	rps/rnds/lps	HrMx%
1			
2			
3			
4			
5			
6			
7			
8			
9			
10			
11			
12			
		A.L.O.I @:	

Ana/Vo2 CARDIO INTERVALS
(Hvi's) mcw est. '13

	Date:	am or pm	Intervals:
	W.O.D.:	rps/rnds/lps	HrMx%
1			
2			
3			
4			
5			
6			
7			
8			
9			
10			
11			
12			
		A.L.O.I @:	

Ana/Vo2 CARDIO INTERVALS
(Hvi's) mcw est. '13

	Date:	am or pm	Intervals:
	W.O.D.:	rps/rnds/lps	HrMx%
1			
2			
3			
4			
5			
6			
7			
8			
9			
10			
11			
12			
		A.L.O.I @:	

Ana/Vo2 CARDIO INTERVALS
(Hvi's) mcw est. '13

	Date:	am or pm	Intervals:
	W.O.D.:	rps/rnds/lps	HrMx%
1			
2			
3			
4			
5			
6			
7			
8			
9			
10			
11			
12			
		A.L.O.I @:	

Ana/Vo2 CARDIO INTERVALS
(Hvi's) mcw est. '13

	Date:	am or pm	Intervals:
	W.O.D.:	rps/rnds/lps	HrMx%
1			
2			
3			
4			
5			
6			
7			
8			
9			
10			
11			
12			
		A.L.O.I @:	

FITNESS EVOLUTION NOTES:

Track your Training Effort Intensity Level Zones, Calorie Expense, and Personal Benchmark Record Data

DATE:________ DATA:	DATE:________ DATA:
DATE:________ DATA:	DATE:________ DATA:
DATE:________ DATA:	DATE:________ DATA:
DATE:________ DATA:	DATE:________ DATA:
DATE:________ DATA:	DATE:________ DATA:
DATE:________ DATA:	DATE:________ DATA:
DATE:________ DATA:	DATE:________ DATA:

FITNESS EVOLUTION NOTES:

Track your Training Effort Intensity Level Zones, Calorie Expense, and Personal Benchmark Record Data

DATE:__________ DATA:	DATE:__________ DATA:
DATE:__________ DATA:	DATE:__________ DATA:
DATE:__________ DATA:	DATE:__________ DATA:
DATE:__________ DATA:	DATE:__________ DATA:
DATE:__________ DATA:	DATE:__________ DATA:
DATE:__________ DATA:	DATE:__________ DATA:
DATE:__________ DATA:	DATE:__________ DATA:

NOTES:

NOTES:

6 Week Training Calendar
Month Year

SUNDAY	MONDAY	TUESDAY	WEDNESDAY	THURSDAY	FRIDAY	SATURDAY

Week 1

Date:	Date:	Date:	Date:	Date:	Date:	Date:
Mileage:	Mileage:	Mileage:	Mileage:	Mileage:	Mileage:	Mileage:

Week 2

Date:	Date:	Date:	Date:	Date:	Date:	Date:
Mileage:	Mileage:	Mileage:	Mileage:	Mileage:	Mileage:	Mileage:

Week 3

Date:	Date:	Date:	Date:	Date:	Date:	Date:
Mileage:	Mileage:	Mileage:	Mileage:	Mileage:	Mileage:	Mileage:

Week 4

Date:	Date:	Date:	Date:	Date:	Date:	Date:
Mileage:	Mileage:	Mileage:	Mileage:	Mileage:	Mileage:	Mileage:

Week 5

Date:	Date:	Date:	Date:	Date:	Date:	Date:
Mileage:	Mileage:	Mileage:	Mileage:	Mileage:	Mileage:	Mileage:

Week 6

Date:	Date:	Date:	Date:	Date:	Date:	Date:
Mileage:	Mileage:	Mileage:	Mileage:	Mileage:	Mileage:	Mileage:

Ana/Vo2 CARDIO INTERVALS
(Hvi's) mcw est. '13

	Date:	am or pm	Intervals:
	W.O.D.:	rps/rnds/lps	HrMx%
1			
2			
3			
4			
5			
6			
7			
8			
9			
10			
11			
12			
		A.L.O.I @:	

Ana/Vo2 CARDIO INTERVALS
(Hvi's) mcw est. '13

	Date:	am or pm	Intervals:
	W.O.D.:	rps/rnds/lps	HrMx%
1			
2			
3			
4			
5			
6			
7			
8			
9			
10			
11			
12			
		A.L.O.I @:	

Ana/Vo2 CARDIO INTERVALS
(Hvi's) mcw est. '13

	Date:	am or pm	Intervals:
	W.O.D.:	rps/rnds/lps	HrMx%
1			
2			
3			
4			
5			
6			
7			
8			
9			
10			
11			
12			
		A.L.O.I @:	

Ana/Vo2 CARDIO INTERVALS
(Hvi's) mcw est. '13

	Date:	am or pm	Intervals:
	W.O.D.:	rps/rnds/lps	HrMx%
1			
2			
3			
4			
5			
6			
7			
8			
9			
10			
11			
12			
		A.L.O.I @:	

Ana/Vo2 CARDIO INTERVALS
(Hvi's) mcw est. '13

	Date:	am or pm	Intervals:
	W.O.D.:	rps/rnds/lps	HrMx%
1			
2			
3			
4			
5			
6			
7			
8			
9			
10			
11			
12			
		A.L.O.I @:	

Ana/Vo2 CARDIO INTERVALS
(Hvi's) mcw est. '13

	Date:	am or pm	Intervals:
	W.O.D.:	rps/rnds/lps	HrMx%
1			
2			
3			
4			
5			
6			
7			
8			
9			
10			
11			
12			
		A.L.O.I @:	

Ana/Vo2 CARDIO INTERVALS

(Hvi's) mcw est. '13

	Date:	am or pm	Intervals:
	W.O.D.:	rps/rnds/lps	HrMx%
1			
2			
3			
4			
5			
6			
7			
8			
9			
10			
11			
12			
		A.L.O.I @:	

Ana/Vo2 CARDIO INTERVALS

(Hvi's) mcw est. '13

	Date:	am or pm	Intervals:
	W.O.D.:	rps/rnds/lps	HrMx%
1			
2			
3			
4			
5			
6			
7			
8			
9			
10			
11			
12			
		A.L.O.I @:	

Ana/Vo2 CARDIO INTERVALS

(Hvi's) mcw est. '13

	Date:	am or pm	Intervals:
	W.O.D.:	rps/rnds/lps	HrMx%
1			
2			
3			
4			
5			
6			
7			
8			
9			
10			
11			
12			
		A.L.O.I @:	

Ana/Vo2 CARDIO INTERVALS

(Hvi's) mcw est. '13

	Date:	am or pm	Intervals:
	W.O.D.:	rps/rnds/lps	HrMx%
1			
2			
3			
4			
5			
6			
7			
8			
9			
10			
11			
12			
		A.L.O.I @:	

Ana/Vo2 CARDIO INTERVALS

(Hvi's) mcw est. '13

	Date:	am or pm	Intervals:
	W.O.D.:	rps/rnds/lps	HrMx%
1			
2			
3			
4			
5			
6			
7			
8			
9			
10			
11			
12			
		A.L.O.I @:	

Ana/Vo2 CARDIO INTERVALS

(Hvi's) mcw est. '13

	Date:	am or pm	Intervals:
	W.O.D.:	rps/rnds/lps	HrMx%
1			
2			
3			
4			
5			
6			
7			
8			
9			
10			
11			
12			
		A.L.O.I @:	

Ana/Vo2 CARDIO INTERVALS
(Hvi's) mcw est. '13

	Date:	am or pm	Intervals:
	W.O.D.:	rps/rnds/lps	HrMx%
1			
2			
3			
4			
5			
6			
7			
8			
9			
10			
11			
12			
		A.L.O.I @:	

Ana/Vo2 CARDIO INTERVALS
(Hvi's) mcw est. '13

	Date:	am or pm	Intervals:
	W.O.D.:	rps/rnds/lps	HrMx%
1			
2			
3			
4			
5			
6			
7			
8			
9			
10			
11			
12			
		A.L.O.I @:	

Ana/Vo2 CARDIO INTERVALS
(Hvi's) mcw est. '13

	Date:	am or pm	Intervals:
	W.O.D.:	rps/rnds/lps	HrMx%
1			
2			
3			
4			
5			
6			
7			
8			
9			
10			
11			
12			
		A.L.O.I @:	

Ana/Vo2 CARDIO INTERVALS
(Hvi's) mcw est. '13

	Date:	am or pm	Intervals:
	W.O.D.:	rps/rnds/lps	HrMx%
1			
2			
3			
4			
5			
6			
7			
8			
9			
10			
11			
12			
		A.L.O.I @:	

Ana/Vo2 CARDIO INTERVALS
(Hvi's) mcw est. '13

	Date:	am or pm	Intervals:
	W.O.D.:	rps/rnds/lps	HrMx%
1			
2			
3			
4			
5			
6			
7			
8			
9			
10			
11			
12			
		A.L.O.I @:	

Ana/Vo2 CARDIO INTERVALS
(Hvi's) mcw est. '13

	Date:	am or pm	Intervals:
	W.O.D.:	rps/rnds/lps	HrMx%
1			
2			
3			
4			
5			
6			
7			
8			
9			
10			
11			
12			
		A.L.O.I @:	

Ana/Vo2 CARDIO INTERVALS
(Hvi's) mcw est. '13

	Date:	am or pm	Intervals:
	W.O.D.:	rps/rnds/lps	HrMx%
1			
2			
3			
4			
5			
6			
7			
8			
9			
10			
11			
12			
		A.L.O.I @:	

Ana/Vo2 CARDIO INTERVALS
(Hvi's) mcw est. '13

	Date:	am or pm	Intervals:
	W.O.D.:	rps/rnds/lps	HrMx%
1			
2			
3			
4			
5			
6			
7			
8			
9			
10			
11			
12			
		A.L.O.I @:	

Ana/Vo2 CARDIO INTERVALS
(Hvi's) mcw est. '13

	Date:	am or pm	Intervals:
	W.O.D.:	rps/rnds/lps	HrMx%
1			
2			
3			
4			
5			
6			
7			
8			
9			
10			
11			
12			
		A.L.O.I @:	

Ana/Vo2 CARDIO INTERVALS
(Hvi's) mcw est. '13

	Date:	am or pm	Intervals:
	W.O.D.:	rps/rnds/lps	HrMx%
1			
2			
3			
4			
5			
6			
7			
8			
9			
10			
11			
12			
		A.L.O.I @:	

Ana/Vo2 CARDIO INTERVALS
(Hvi's) mcw est. '13

	Date:	am or pm	Intervals:
	W.O.D.:	rps/rnds/lps	HrMx%
1			
2			
3			
4			
5			
6			
7			
8			
9			
10			
11			
12			
		A.L.O.I @:	

Ana/Vo2 CARDIO INTERVALS
(Hvi's) mcw est. '13

	Date:	am or pm	Intervals:
	W.O.D.:	rps/rnds/lps	HrMx%
1			
2			
3			
4			
5			
6			
7			
8			
9			
10			
11			
12			
		A.L.O.I @:	

Ana/Vo2 CARDIO INTERVALS
(Hvi's) mcw est. '13

	Date:	am or pm	Intervals:
	W.O.D.:	rps/rnds/lps	HrMx%
1			
2			
3			
4			
5			
6			
7			
8			
9			
10			
11			
12			
		A.L.O.I @:	

Ana/Vo2 CARDIO INTERVALS
(Hvi's) mcw est. '13

	Date:	am or pm	Intervals:
	W.O.D.:	rps/rnds/lps	HrMx%
1			
2			
3			
4			
5			
6			
7			
8			
9			
10			
11			
12			
		A.L.O.I @:	

Ana/Vo2 CARDIO INTERVALS
(Hvi's) mcw est. '13

	Date:	am or pm	Intervals:
	W.O.D.:	rps/rnds/lps	HrMx%
1			
2			
3			
4			
5			
6			
7			
8			
9			
10			
11			
12			
		A.L.O.I @:	

Ana/Vo2 CARDIO INTERVALS
(Hvi's) mcw est. '13

	Date:	am or pm	Intervals:
	W.O.D.:	rps/rnds/lps	HrMx%
1			
2			
3			
4			
5			
6			
7			
8			
9			
10			
11			
12			
		A.L.O.I @:	

Ana/Vo2 CARDIO INTERVALS
(Hvi's) mcw est. '13

	Date:	am or pm	Intervals:
	W.O.D.:	rps/rnds/lps	HrMx%
1			
2			
3			
4			
5			
6			
7			
8			
9			
10			
11			
12			
		A.L.O.I @:	

Ana/Vo2 CARDIO INTERVALS
(Hvi's) mcw est. '13

	Date:	am or pm	Intervals:
	W.O.D.:	rps/rnds/lps	HrMx%
1			
2			
3			
4			
5			
6			
7			
8			
9			
10			
11			
12			
		A.L.O.I @:	

FITNESS EVOLUTION NOTES:

Track your Training Effort Intensity Level Zones, Calorie Expense, and Personal Benchmark Record Data

DATE:__________ DATA:	DATE:__________ DATA:
DATE:__________ DATA:	DATE:__________ DATA:
DATE:__________ DATA:	DATE:__________ DATA:
DATE:__________ DATA:	DATE:__________ DATA:
DATE:__________ DATA:	DATE:__________ DATA:
DATE:__________ DATA:	DATE:__________ DATA:
DATE:__________ DATA:	DATE:__________ DATA:

FITNESS EVOLUTION NOTES:

Track your Training Effort Intensity Level Zones, Calorie Expense, and Personal Benchmark Record Data

DATE:_______ DATA:	DATE:_______ DATA:
DATE:_______ DATA:	DATE:_______ DATA:
DATE:_______ DATA:	DATE:_______ DATA:
DATE:_______ DATA:	DATE:_______ DATA:
DATE:_______ DATA:	DATE:_______ DATA:
DATE:_______ DATA:	DATE:_______ DATA:
DATE:_______ DATA:	DATE:_______ DATA:

NOTES:

NOTES:

6 Week Training Calendar
Month Year

SUNDAY	MONDAY	TUESDAY	WEDNESDAY	THURSDAY	FRIDAY	SATURDAY

Week 1

Date:	Date:	Date:	Date:	Date:	Date:	Date:
Mileage:	Mileage:	Mileage:	Mileage:	Mileage:	Mileage:	Mileage:

Week 2

Date:	Date:	Date:	Date:	Date:	Date:	Date:
Mileage:	Mileage:	Mileage:	Mileage:	Mileage:	Mileage:	Mileage:

Week 3

Date:	Date:	Date:	Date:	Date:	Date:	Date:
Mileage:	Mileage:	Mileage:	Mileage:	Mileage:	Mileage:	Mileage:

Week 4

Date:	Date:	Date:	Date:	Date:	Date:	Date:
Mileage:	Mileage:	Mileage:	Mileage:	Mileage:	Mileage:	Mileage:

Week 5

Date:	Date:	Date:	Date:	Date:	Date:	Date:
Mileage:	Mileage:	Mileage:	Mileage:	Mileage:	Mileage:	Mileage:

Week 6

Date:	Date:	Date:	Date:	Date:	Date:	Date:
Mileage:	Mileage:	Mileage:	Mileage:	Mileage:	Mileage:	Mileage:

Ana/Vo2 CARDIO INTERVALS
(Hvi's) mcw est. '13

	Date:	am or pm	Intervals:
	W.O.D.:	rps/rnds/lps	HrMx%
1			
2			
3			
4			
5			
6			
7			
8			
9			
10			
11			
12			
		A.L.O.I @:	

Ana/Vo2 CARDIO INTERVALS
(Hvi's) mcw est. '13

	Date:	am or pm	Intervals:
	W.O.D.:	rps/rnds/lps	HrMx%
1			
2			
3			
4			
5			
6			
7			
8			
9			
10			
11			
12			
		A.L.O.I @:	

Ana/Vo2 CARDIO INTERVALS
(Hvi's) mcw est. '13

	Date:	am or pm	Intervals:
	W.O.D.:	rps/rnds/lps	HrMx%
1			
2			
3			
4			
5			
6			
7			
8			
9			
10			
11			
12			
		A.L.O.I @:	

Ana/Vo2 CARDIO INTERVALS
(Hvi's) mcw est. '13

	Date:	am or pm	Intervals:
	W.O.D.:	rps/rnds/lps	HrMx%
1			
2			
3			
4			
5			
6			
7			
8			
9			
10			
11			
12			
		A.L.O.I @:	

Ana/Vo2 CARDIO INTERVALS
(Hvi's) mcw est. '13

	Date:	am or pm	Intervals:
	W.O.D.:	rps/rnds/lps	HrMx%
1			
2			
3			
4			
5			
6			
7			
8			
9			
10			
11			
12			
		A.L.O.I @:	

Ana/Vo2 CARDIO INTERVALS
(Hvi's) mcw est. '13

	Date:	am or pm	Intervals:
	W.O.D.:	rps/rnds/lps	HrMx%
1			
2			
3			
4			
5			
6			
7			
8			
9			
10			
11			
12			
		A.L.O.I @:	

Ana/Vo2 CARDIO INTERVALS
(Hvi's) mcw est. '13

	Date:	am or pm	Intervals:
	W.O.D.:	rps/rnds/lps	HrMx%
1			
2			
3			
4			
5			
6			
7			
8			
9			
10			
11			
12			
		A.L.O.I @:	

Ana/Vo2 CARDIO INTERVALS
(Hvi's) mcw est. '13

	Date:	am or pm	Intervals:
	W.O.D.:	rps/rnds/lps	HrMx%
1			
2			
3			
4			
5			
6			
7			
8			
9			
10			
11			
12			
		A.L.O.I @:	

Ana/Vo2 CARDIO INTERVALS
(Hvi's) mcw est. '13

	Date:	am or pm	Intervals:
	W.O.D.:	rps/rnds/lps	HrMx%
1			
2			
3			
4			
5			
6			
7			
8			
9			
10			
11			
12			
		A.L.O.I @:	

Ana/Vo2 CARDIO INTERVALS
(Hvi's) mcw est. '13

	Date:	am or pm	Intervals:
	W.O.D.:	rps/rnds/lps	HrMx%
1			
2			
3			
4			
5			
6			
7			
8			
9			
10			
11			
12			
		A.L.O.I @:	

Ana/Vo2 CARDIO INTERVALS
(Hvi's) mcw est. '13

	Date:	am or pm	Intervals:
	W.O.D.:	rps/rnds/lps	HrMx%
1			
2			
3			
4			
5			
6			
7			
8			
9			
10			
11			
12			
		A.L.O.I @:	

Ana/Vo2 CARDIO INTERVALS
(Hvi's) mcw est. '13

	Date:	am or pm	Intervals:
	W.O.D.:	rps/rnds/lps	HrMx%
1			
2			
3			
4			
5			
6			
7			
8			
9			
10			
11			
12			
		A.L.O.I @:	

Ana/Vo2 CARDIO INTERVALS

(Hvi's) mcw est. '13

	Date:	am or pm	Intervals:
	W.O.D.:	rps/rnds/lps	HrMx%
1			
2			
3			
4			
5			
6			
7			
8			
9			
10			
11			
12			
		A.L.O.I @:	

Ana/Vo2 CARDIO INTERVALS

(Hvi's) mcw est. '13

	Date:	am or pm	Intervals:
	W.O.D.:	rps/rnds/lps	HrMx%
1			
2			
3			
4			
5			
6			
7			
8			
9			
10			
11			
12			
		A.L.O.I @:	

Ana/Vo2 CARDIO INTERVALS

(Hvi's) mcw est. '13

	Date:	am or pm	Intervals:
	W.O.D.:	rps/rnds/lps	HrMx%
1			
2			
3			
4			
5			
6			
7			
8			
9			
10			
11			
12			
		A.L.O.I @:	

Ana/Vo2 CARDIO INTERVALS

(Hvi's) mcw est. '13

	Date:	am or pm	Intervals:
	W.O.D.:	rps/rnds/lps	HrMx%
1			
2			
3			
4			
5			
6			
7			
8			
9			
10			
11			
12			
		A.L.O.I @:	

Ana/Vo2 CARDIO INTERVALS

(Hvi's) mcw est. '13

	Date:	am or pm	Intervals:
	W.O.D.:	rps/rnds/lps	HrMx%
1			
2			
3			
4			
5			
6			
7			
8			
9			
10			
11			
12			
		A.L.O.I @:	

Ana/Vo2 CARDIO INTERVALS

(Hvi's) mcw est. '13

	Date:	am or pm	Intervals:
	W.O.D.:	rps/rnds/lps	HrMx%
1			
2			
3			
4			
5			
6			
7			
8			
9			
10			
11			
12			
		A.L.O.I @:	

Ana/Vo2 CARDIO INTERVALS

(Hvi's) mcw est. '13

	Date:	am or pm	Intervals:
	W.O.D.:	rps/rnds/lps	HrMx%
1			
2			
3			
4			
5			
6			
7			
8			
9			
10			
11			
12			
		A.L.O.I @:	

Ana/Vo2 CARDIO INTERVALS

(Hvi's) mcw est. '13

	Date:	am or pm	Intervals:
	W.O.D.:	rps/rnds/lps	HrMx%
1			
2			
3			
4			
5			
6			
7			
8			
9			
10			
11			
12			
		A.L.O.I @:	

Ana/Vo2 CARDIO INTERVALS

(Hvi's) mcw est. '13

	Date:	am or pm	Intervals:
	W.O.D.:	rps/rnds/lps	HrMx%
1			
2			
3			
4			
5			
6			
7			
8			
9			
10			
11			
12			
		A.L.O.I @:	

Ana/Vo2 CARDIO INTERVALS

(Hvi's) mcw est. '13

	Date:	am or pm	Intervals:
	W.O.D.:	rps/rnds/lps	HrMx%
1			
2			
3			
4			
5			
6			
7			
8			
9			
10			
11			
12			
		A.L.O.I @:	

Ana/Vo2 CARDIO INTERVALS

(Hvi's) mcw est. '13

	Date:	am or pm	Intervals:
	W.O.D.:	rps/rnds/lps	HrMx%
1			
2			
3			
4			
5			
6			
7			
8			
9			
10			
11			
12			
		A.L.O.I @:	

Ana/Vo2 CARDIO INTERVALS

(Hvi's) mcw est. '13

	Date:	am or pm	Intervals:
	W.O.D.:	rps/rnds/lps	HrMx%
1			
2			
3			
4			
5			
6			
7			
8			
9			
10			
11			
12			
		A.L.O.I @:	

Ana/Vo2 CARDIO INTERVALS
(Hvi's) mcw est. '13

	Date:	am or pm	Intervals:
	W.O.D.:	rps/rnds/lps	HrMx%
1			
2			
3			
4			
5			
6			
7			
8			
9			
10			
11			
12			
		A.L.O.I @:	

Ana/Vo2 CARDIO INTERVALS
(Hvi's) mcw est. '13

	Date:	am or pm	Intervals:
	W.O.D.:	rps/rnds/lps	HrMx%
1			
2			
3			
4			
5			
6			
7			
8			
9			
10			
11			
12			
		A.L.O.I @:	

Ana/Vo2 CARDIO INTERVALS
(Hvi's) mcw est. '13

	Date:	am or pm	Intervals:
	W.O.D.:	rps/rnds/lps	HrMx%
1			
2			
3			
4			
5			
6			
7			
8			
9			
10			
11			
12			
		A.L.O.I @:	

Ana/Vo2 CARDIO INTERVALS
(Hvi's) mcw est. '13

	Date:	am or pm	Intervals:
	W.O.D.:	rps/rnds/lps	HrMx%
1			
2			
3			
4			
5			
6			
7			
8			
9			
10			
11			
12			
		A.L.O.I @:	

Ana/Vo2 CARDIO INTERVALS
(Hvi's) mcw est. '13

	Date:	am or pm	Intervals:
	W.O.D.:	rps/rnds/lps	HrMx%
1			
2			
3			
4			
5			
6			
7			
8			
9			
10			
11			
12			
		A.L.O.I @:	

Ana/Vo2 CARDIO INTERVALS
(Hvi's) mcw est. '13

	Date:	am or pm	Intervals:
	W.O.D.:	rps/rnds/lps	HrMx%
1			
2			
3			
4			
5			
6			
7			
8			
9			
10			
11			
12			
		A.L.O.I @:	

FITNESS EVOLUTION NOTES:

Track your Training Effort Intensity Level Zones, Calorie Expense, and Personal Benchmark Record Data

DATE:________ DATA:	DATE:________ DATA:
DATE:________ DATA:	DATE:________ DATA:
DATE:________ DATA:	DATE:________ DATA:
DATE:________ DATA:	DATE:________ DATA:
DATE:________ DATA:	DATE:________ DATA:
DATE:________ DATA:	DATE:________ DATA:
DATE:________ DATA:	DATE:________ DATA:

FITNESS EVOLUTION NOTES:

Track your Training Effort Intensity Level Zones, Calorie Expense, and Personal Benchmark Record Data

DATE:__________ DATA:	DATE:__________ DATA:
DATE:__________ DATA:	DATE:__________ DATA:
DATE:__________ DATA:	DATE:__________ DATA:
DATE:__________ DATA:	DATE:__________ DATA:
DATE:__________ DATA:	DATE:__________ DATA:
DATE:__________ DATA:	DATE:__________ DATA:
DATE:__________ DATA:	DATE:__________ DATA:

NOTES:

NOTES:

6 Week Training Calendar

Month Year

SUNDAY	MONDAY	TUESDAY	WEDNESDAY	THURSDAY	FRIDAY	SATURDAY

Week 1

Date:	Date:	Date:	Date:	Date:	Date:	Date:
Mileage:	Mileage:	Mileage:	Mileage:	Mileage:	Mileage:	Mileage:

Week 2

Date:	Date:	Date:	Date:	Date:	Date:	Date:
Mileage:	Mileage:	Mileage:	Mileage:	Mileage:	Mileage:	Mileage:

Week 3

Date:	Date:	Date:	Date:	Date:	Date:	Date:
Mileage:	Mileage:	Mileage:	Mileage:	Mileage:	Mileage:	Mileage:

Week 4

Date:	Date:	Date:	Date:	Date:	Date:	Date:
Mileage:	Mileage:	Mileage:	Mileage:	Mileage:	Mileage:	Mileage:

Week 5

Date:	Date:	Date:	Date:	Date:	Date:	Date:
Mileage:	Mileage:	Mileage:	Mileage:	Mileage:	Mileage:	Mileage:

Week 6

Date:	Date:	Date:	Date:	Date:	Date:	Date:
Mileage:	Mileage:	Mileage:	Mileage:	Mileage:	Mileage:	Mileage:

Ana/Vo2 CARDIO INTERVALS
(Hvi's) mcw est. '13

	Date:	am or pm	Intervals:
	W.O.D.:	rps/rnds/lps	HrMx%
1			
2			
3			
4			
5			
6			
7			
8			
9			
10			
11			
12			
		A.L.O.I @:	

Ana/Vo2 CARDIO INTERVALS
(Hvi's) mcw est. '13

	Date:	am or pm	Intervals:
	W.O.D.:	rps/rnds/lps	HrMx%
1			
2			
3			
4			
5			
6			
7			
8			
9			
10			
11			
12			
		A.L.O.I @:	

Ana/Vo2 CARDIO INTERVALS
(Hvi's) mcw est. '13

	Date:	am or pm	Intervals:
	W.O.D.:	rps/rnds/lps	HrMx%
1			
2			
3			
4			
5			
6			
7			
8			
9			
10			
11			
12			
		A.L.O.I @:	

Ana/Vo2 CARDIO INTERVALS
(Hvi's) mcw est. '13

	Date:	am or pm	Intervals:
	W.O.D.:	rps/rnds/lps	HrMx%
1			
2			
3			
4			
5			
6			
7			
8			
9			
10			
11			
12			
		A.L.O.I @:	

Ana/Vo2 CARDIO INTERVALS
(Hvi's) mcw est. '13

	Date:	am or pm	Intervals:
	W.O.D.:	rps/rnds/lps	HrMx%
1			
2			
3			
4			
5			
6			
7			
8			
9			
10			
11			
12			
		A.L.O.I @:	

Ana/Vo2 CARDIO INTERVALS
(Hvi's) mcw est. '13

	Date:	am or pm	Intervals:
	W.O.D.:	rps/rnds/lps	HrMx%
1			
2			
3			
4			
5			
6			
7			
8			
9			
10			
11			
12			
		A.L.O.I @:	

Ana/Vo2 CARDIO INTERVALS
(Hvi's) mcw est. '13

	Date:	am or pm	Intervals:
	W.O.D.:	rps/rnds/lps	HrMx%
1			
2			
3			
4			
5			
6			
7			
8			
9			
10			
11			
12			
		A.L.O.I @:	

Ana/Vo2 CARDIO INTERVALS
(Hvi's) mcw est. '13

	Date:	am or pm	Intervals:
	W.O.D.:	rps/rnds/lps	HrMx%
1			
2			
3			
4			
5			
6			
7			
8			
9			
10			
11			
12			
		A.L.O.I @:	

Ana/Vo2 CARDIO INTERVALS
(Hvi's) mcw est. '13

	Date:	am or pm	Intervals:
	W.O.D.:	rps/rnds/lps	HrMx%
1			
2			
3			
4			
5			
6			
7			
8			
9			
10			
11			
12			
		A.L.O.I @:	

Ana/Vo2 CARDIO INTERVALS
(Hvi's) mcw est. '13

	Date:	am or pm	Intervals:
	W.O.D.:	rps/rnds/lps	HrMx%
1			
2			
3			
4			
5			
6			
7			
8			
9			
10			
11			
12			
		A.L.O.I @:	

Ana/Vo2 CARDIO INTERVALS
(Hvi's) mcw est. '13

	Date:	am or pm	Intervals:
	W.O.D.:	rps/rnds/lps	HrMx%
1			
2			
3			
4			
5			
6			
7			
8			
9			
10			
11			
12			
		A.L.O.I @:	

Ana/Vo2 CARDIO INTERVALS
(Hvi's) mcw est. '13

	Date:	am or pm	Intervals:
	W.O.D.:	rps/rnds/lps	HrMx%
1			
2			
3			
4			
5			
6			
7			
8			
9			
10			
11			
12			
		A.L.O.I @:	

Ana/Vo2 CARDIO INTERVALS
(Hvi's) mcw est. '13

	Date:	am or pm	Intervals:
	W.O.D.:	rps/rnds/lps	HrMx%
1			
2			
3			
4			
5			
6			
7			
8			
9			
10			
11			
12			
		A.L.O.I @:	

Ana/Vo2 CARDIO INTERVALS
(Hvi's) mcw est. '13

	Date:	am or pm	Intervals:
	W.O.D.:	rps/rnds/lps	HrMx%
1			
2			
3			
4			
5			
6			
7			
8			
9			
10			
11			
12			
		A.L.O.I @:	

Ana/Vo2 CARDIO INTERVALS
(Hvi's) mcw est. '13

	Date:	am or pm	Intervals:
	W.O.D.:	rps/rnds/lps	HrMx%
1			
2			
3			
4			
5			
6			
7			
8			
9			
10			
11			
12			
		A.L.O.I @:	

Ana/Vo2 CARDIO INTERVALS
(Hvi's) mcw est. '13

	Date:	am or pm	Intervals:
	W.O.D.:	rps/rnds/lps	HrMx%
1			
2			
3			
4			
5			
6			
7			
8			
9			
10			
11			
12			
		A.L.O.I @:	

Ana/Vo2 CARDIO INTERVALS
(Hvi's) mcw est. '13

	Date:	am or pm	Intervals:
	W.O.D.:	rps/rnds/lps	HrMx%
1			
2			
3			
4			
5			
6			
7			
8			
9			
10			
11			
12			
		A.L.O.I @:	

Ana/Vo2 CARDIO INTERVALS
(Hvi's) mcw est. '13

	Date:	am or pm	Intervals:
	W.O.D.:	rps/rnds/lps	HrMx%
1			
2			
3			
4			
5			
6			
7			
8			
9			
10			
11			
12			
		A.L.O.I @:	

Ana/Vo2 CARDIO INTERVALS

(Hvi's) mcw est. '13

	Date:	am or pm	Intervals:
	W.O.D.:	rps/rnds/lps	HrMx%
1			
2			
3			
4			
5			
6			
7			
8			
9			
10			
11			
12			
		A.L.O.I @:	

Ana/Vo2 CARDIO INTERVALS

(Hvi's) mcw est. '13

	Date:	am or pm	Intervals:
	W.O.D.:	rps/rnds/lps	HrMx%
1			
2			
3			
4			
5			
6			
7			
8			
9			
10			
11			
12			
		A.L.O.I @:	

Ana/Vo2 CARDIO INTERVALS

(Hvi's) mcw est. '13

	Date:	am or pm	Intervals:
	W.O.D.:	rps/rnds/lps	HrMx%
1			
2			
3			
4			
5			
6			
7			
8			
9			
10			
11			
12			
		A.L.O.I @:	

Ana/Vo2 CARDIO INTERVALS

(Hvi's) mcw est. '13

	Date:	am or pm	Intervals:
	W.O.D.:	rps/rnds/lps	HrMx%
1			
2			
3			
4			
5			
6			
7			
8			
9			
10			
11			
12			
		A.L.O.I @:	

Ana/Vo2 CARDIO INTERVALS

(Hvi's) mcw est. '13

	Date:	am or pm	Intervals:
	W.O.D.:	rps/rnds/lps	HrMx%
1			
2			
3			
4			
5			
6			
7			
8			
9			
10			
11			
12			
		A.L.O.I @:	

Ana/Vo2 CARDIO INTERVALS

(Hvi's) mcw est. '13

	Date:	am or pm	Intervals:
	W.O.D.:	rps/rnds/lps	HrMx%
1			
2			
3			
4			
5			
6			
7			
8			
9			
10			
11			
12			
		A.L.O.I @:	

Ana/Vo2 CARDIO INTERVALS
(Hvi's) mcw est. '13

	Date:	am or pm	Intervals:
	W.O.D.:	rps/rnds/lps	HrMx%
1			
2			
3			
4			
5			
6			
7			
8			
9			
10			
11			
12			
		A.L.O.I @:	

Ana/Vo2 CARDIO INTERVALS
(Hvi's) mcw est. '13

	Date:	am or pm	Intervals:
	W.O.D.:	rps/rnds/lps	HrMx%
1			
2			
3			
4			
5			
6			
7			
8			
9			
10			
11			
12			
		A.L.O.I @:	

Ana/Vo2 CARDIO INTERVALS
(Hvi's) mcw est. '13

	Date:	am or pm	Intervals:
	W.O.D.:	rps/rnds/lps	HrMx%
1			
2			
3			
4			
5			
6			
7			
8			
9			
10			
11			
12			
		A.L.O.I @:	

Ana/Vo2 CARDIO INTERVALS
(Hvi's) mcw est. '13

	Date:	am or pm	Intervals:
	W.O.D.:	rps/rnds/lps	HrMx%
1			
2			
3			
4			
5			
6			
7			
8			
9			
10			
11			
12			
		A.L.O.I @:	

Ana/Vo2 CARDIO INTERVALS
(Hvi's) mcw est. '13

	Date:	am or pm	Intervals:
	W.O.D.:	rps/rnds/lps	HrMx%
1			
2			
3			
4			
5			
6			
7			
8			
9			
10			
11			
12			
		A.L.O.I @:	

Ana/Vo2 CARDIO INTERVALS
(Hvi's) mcw est. '13

	Date:	am or pm	Intervals:
	W.O.D.:	rps/rnds/lps	HrMx%
1			
2			
3			
4			
5			
6			
7			
8			
9			
10			
11			
12			
		A.L.O.I @:	

FITNESS EVOLUTION NOTES:

Track your Training Effort Intensity Level Zones, Calorie Expense, and Personal Benchmark Record Data

DATE:________ DATA:	DATE:________ DATA:
DATE:________ DATA:	DATE:________ DATA:
DATE:________ DATA:	DATE:________ DATA:
DATE:________ DATA:	DATE:________ DATA:
DATE:________ DATA:	DATE:________ DATA:
DATE:________ DATA:	DATE:________ DATA:
DATE:________ DATA:	DATE:________ DATA:

FITNESS EVOLUTION NOTES:

Track your Training Effort Intensity Level Zones, Calorie Expense, and Personal Benchmark Record Data

DATE:__________ DATA:	DATE:__________ DATA:
DATE:__________ DATA:	DATE:__________ DATA:
DATE:__________ DATA:	DATE:__________ DATA:
DATE:__________ DATA:	DATE:__________ DATA:
DATE:__________ DATA:	DATE:__________ DATA:
DATE:__________ DATA:	DATE:__________ DATA:
DATE:__________ DATA:	DATE:__________ DATA:

NOTES:

NOTES:

6 Week Training Calendar

Month Year

SUNDAY	MONDAY	TUESDAY	WEDNESDAY	THURSDAY	FRIDAY	SATURDAY

Week 1

Date:	Date:	Date:	Date:	Date:	Date:	Date:
Mileage:	Mileage:	Mileage:	Mileage:	Mileage:	Mileage:	Mileage:

Week 2

Date:	Date:	Date:	Date:	Date:	Date:	Date:
Mileage:	Mileage:	Mileage:	Mileage:	Mileage:	Mileage:	Mileage:

Week 3

Date:	Date:	Date:	Date:	Date:	Date:	Date:
Mileage:	Mileage:	Mileage:	Mileage:	Mileage:	Mileage:	Mileage:

Week 4

Date:	Date:	Date:	Date:	Date:	Date:	Date:
Mileage:	Mileage:	Mileage:	Mileage:	Mileage:	Mileage:	Mileage:

Week 5

Date:	Date:	Date:	Date:	Date:	Date:	Date:
Mileage:	Mileage:	Mileage:	Mileage:	Mileage:	Mileage:	Mileage:

Week 6

Date:	Date:	Date:	Date:	Date:	Date:	Date:
Mileage:	Mileage:	Mileage:	Mileage:	Mileage:	Mileage:	Mileage:

Ana/Vo2 CARDIO INTERVALS

(Hvi's) mcw est. '13

	Date:	am or pm	Intervals:
	W.O.D.:	rps/rnds/lps	HrMx%
1			
2			
3			
4			
5			
6			
7			
8			
9			
10			
11			
12			
		A.L.O.I @:	

Ana/Vo2 CARDIO INTERVALS

(Hvi's) mcw est. '13

	Date:	am or pm	Intervals:
	W.O.D.:	rps/rnds/lps	HrMx%
1			
2			
3			
4			
5			
6			
7			
8			
9			
10			
11			
12			
		A.L.O.I @:	

Ana/Vo2 CARDIO INTERVALS

(Hvi's) mcw est. '13

	Date:	am or pm	Intervals:
	W.O.D.:	rps/rnds/lps	HrMx%
1			
2			
3			
4			
5			
6			
7			
8			
9			
10			
11			
12			
		A.L.O.I @:	

Ana/Vo2 CARDIO INTERVALS

(Hvi's) mcw est. '13

	Date:	am or pm	Intervals:
	W.O.D.:	rps/rnds/lps	HrMx%
1			
2			
3			
4			
5			
6			
7			
8			
9			
10			
11			
12			
		A.L.O.I @:	

Ana/Vo2 CARDIO INTERVALS

(Hvi's) mcw est. '13

	Date:	am or pm	Intervals:
	W.O.D.:	rps/rnds/lps	HrMx%
1			
2			
3			
4			
5			
6			
7			
8			
9			
10			
11			
12			
		A.L.O.I @:	

Ana/Vo2 CARDIO INTERVALS

(Hvi's) mcw est. '13

	Date:	am or pm	Intervals:
	W.O.D.:	rps/rnds/lps	HrMx%
1			
2			
3			
4			
5			
6			
7			
8			
9			
10			
11			
12			
		A.L.O.I @:	

Ana/Vo2 CARDIO INTERVALS
(Hvi's) mcw est. '13

	Date:	am or pm	Intervals:
	W.O.D.:	rps/rnds/lps	HrMx%
1			
2			
3			
4			
5			
6			
7			
8			
9			
10			
11			
12			
		A.L.O.I @:	

Ana/Vo2 CARDIO INTERVALS
(Hvi's) mcw est. '13

	Date:	am or pm	Intervals:
	W.O.D.:	rps/rnds/lps	HrMx%
1			
2			
3			
4			
5			
6			
7			
8			
9			
10			
11			
12			
		A.L.O.I @:	

Ana/Vo2 CARDIO INTERVALS
(Hvi's) mcw est. '13

	Date:	am or pm	Intervals:
	W.O.D.:	rps/rnds/lps	HrMx%
1			
2			
3			
4			
5			
6			
7			
8			
9			
10			
11			
12			
		A.L.O.I @:	

Ana/Vo2 CARDIO INTERVALS
(Hvi's) mcw est. '13

	Date:	am or pm	Intervals:
	W.O.D.:	rps/rnds/lps	HrMx%
1			
2			
3			
4			
5			
6			
7			
8			
9			
10			
11			
12			
		A.L.O.I @:	

Ana/Vo2 CARDIO INTERVALS
(Hvi's) mcw est. '13

	Date:	am or pm	Intervals:
	W.O.D.:	rps/rnds/lps	HrMx%
1			
2			
3			
4			
5			
6			
7			
8			
9			
10			
11			
12			
		A.L.O.I @:	

Ana/Vo2 CARDIO INTERVALS
(Hvi's) mcw est. '13

	Date:	am or pm	Intervals:
	W.O.D.:	rps/rnds/lps	HrMx%
1			
2			
3			
4			
5			
6			
7			
8			
9			
10			
11			
12			
		A.L.O.I @:	

Ana/Vo2 CARDIO INTERVALS

(Hvi's) mcw est. '13

	Date:	am or pm	Intervals:
	W.O.D.:	rps/rnds/lps	HrMx%
1			
2			
3			
4			
5			
6			
7			
8			
9			
10			
11			
12			
		A.L.O.I @:	

Ana/Vo2 CARDIO INTERVALS

(Hvi's) mcw est. '13

	Date:	am or pm	Intervals:
	W.O.D.:	rps/rnds/lps	HrMx%
1			
2			
3			
4			
5			
6			
7			
8			
9			
10			
11			
12			
		A.L.O.I @:	

Ana/Vo2 CARDIO INTERVALS

(Hvi's) mcw est. '13

	Date:	am or pm	Intervals:
	W.O.D.:	rps/rnds/lps	HrMx%
1			
2			
3			
4			
5			
6			
7			
8			
9			
10			
11			
12			
		A.L.O.I @:	

Ana/Vo2 CARDIO INTERVALS

(Hvi's) mcw est. '13

	Date:	am or pm	Intervals:
	W.O.D.:	rps/rnds/lps	HrMx%
1			
2			
3			
4			
5			
6			
7			
8			
9			
10			
11			
12			
		A.L.O.I @:	

Ana/Vo2 CARDIO INTERVALS

(Hvi's) mcw est. '13

	Date:	am or pm	Intervals:
	W.O.D.:	rps/rnds/lps	HrMx%
1			
2			
3			
4			
5			
6			
7			
8			
9			
10			
11			
12			
		A.L.O.I @:	

Ana/Vo2 CARDIO INTERVALS

(Hvi's) mcw est. '13

	Date:	am or pm	Intervals:
	W.O.D.:	rps/rnds/lps	HrMx%
1			
2			
3			
4			
5			
6			
7			
8			
9			
10			
11			
12			
		A.L.O.I @:	

Ana/Vo2 CARDIO INTERVALS
(Hvi's) mcw est. '13

	Date:	am or pm	Intervals:
	W.O.D.:	rps/rnds/lps	HrMx%
1			
2			
3			
4			
5			
6			
7			
8			
9			
10			
11			
12			
		A.L.O.I @:	

Ana/Vo2 CARDIO INTERVALS
(Hvi's) mcw est. '13

	Date:	am or pm	Intervals:
	W.O.D.:	rps/rnds/lps	HrMx%
1			
2			
3			
4			
5			
6			
7			
8			
9			
10			
11			
12			
		A.L.O.I @:	

Ana/Vo2 CARDIO INTERVALS
(Hvi's) mcw est. '13

	Date:	am or pm	Intervals:
	W.O.D.:	rps/rnds/lps	HrMx%
1			
2			
3			
4			
5			
6			
7			
8			
9			
10			
11			
12			
		A.L.O.I @:	

Ana/Vo2 CARDIO INTERVALS
(Hvi's) mcw est. '13

	Date:	am or pm	Intervals:
	W.O.D.:	rps/rnds/lps	HrMx%
1			
2			
3			
4			
5			
6			
7			
8			
9			
10			
11			
12			
		A.L.O.I @:	

Ana/Vo2 CARDIO INTERVALS
(Hvi's) mcw est. '13

	Date:	am or pm	Intervals:
	W.O.D.:	rps/rnds/lps	HrMx%
1			
2			
3			
4			
5			
6			
7			
8			
9			
10			
11			
12			
		A.L.O.I @:	

Ana/Vo2 CARDIO INTERVALS
(Hvi's) mcw est. '13

	Date:	am or pm	Intervals:
	W.O.D.:	rps/rnds/lps	HrMx%
1			
2			
3			
4			
5			
6			
7			
8			
9			
10			
11			
12			
		A.L.O.I @:	

Ana/Vo2 CARDIO INTERVALS

(Hvi's) mcw est. '13

	Date:	am or pm	Intervals:
	W.O.D.:	rps/rnds/lps	HrMx%
1			
2			
3			
4			
5			
6			
7			
8			
9			
10			
11			
12			
		A.L.O.I @:	

Ana/Vo2 CARDIO INTERVALS

(Hvi's) mcw est. '13

	Date:	am or pm	Intervals:
	W.O.D.:	rps/rnds/lps	HrMx%
1			
2			
3			
4			
5			
6			
7			
8			
9			
10			
11			
12			
		A.L.O.I @:	

Ana/Vo2 CARDIO INTERVALS

(Hvi's) mcw est. '13

	Date:	am or pm	Intervals:
	W.O.D.:	rps/rnds/lps	HrMx%
1			
2			
3			
4			
5			
6			
7			
8			
9			
10			
11			
12			
		A.L.O.I @:	

Ana/Vo2 CARDIO INTERVALS

(Hvi's) mcw est. '13

	Date:	am or pm	Intervals:
	W.O.D.:	rps/rnds/lps	HrMx%
1			
2			
3			
4			
5			
6			
7			
8			
9			
10			
11			
12			
		A.L.O.I @:	

Ana/Vo2 CARDIO INTERVALS

(Hvi's) mcw est. '13

	Date:	am or pm	Intervals:
	W.O.D.:	rps/rnds/lps	HrMx%
1			
2			
3			
4			
5			
6			
7			
8			
9			
10			
11			
12			
		A.L.O.I @:	

Ana/Vo2 CARDIO INTERVALS

(Hvi's) mcw est. '13

	Date:	am or pm	Intervals:
	W.O.D.:	rps/rnds/lps	HrMx%
1			
2			
3			
4			
5			
6			
7			
8			
9			
10			
11			
12			
		A.L.O.I @:	

FITNESS EVOLUTION NOTES:

Track your Training Effort Intensity Level Zones, Calorie Expense, and Personal Benchmark Record Data

DATE:______ DATA:	DATE:______ DATA:
DATE:______ DATA:	DATE:______ DATA:
DATE:______ DATA:	DATE:______ DATA:
DATE:______ DATA:	DATE:______ DATA:
DATE:______ DATA:	DATE:______ DATA:
DATE:______ DATA:	DATE:______ DATA:
DATE:______ DATA:	DATE:______ DATA:

FITNESS EVOLUTION NOTES:

Track your Training Effort Intensity Level Zones, Calorie Expense, and Personal Benchmark Record Data

DATE:________ DATA:	DATE:________ DATA:
DATE:________ DATA:	DATE:________ DATA:
DATE:________ DATA:	DATE:________ DATA:
DATE:________ DATA:	DATE:________ DATA:
DATE:________ DATA:	DATE:________ DATA:
DATE:________ DATA:	DATE:________ DATA:
DATE:________ DATA:	DATE:________ DATA:

NOTES:

NOTES:

6 Week Training Calendar

Month Year

SUNDAY	MONDAY	TUESDAY	WEDNESDAY	THURSDAY	FRIDAY	SATURDAY

Week 1

Date:	Date:	Date:	Date:	Date:	Date:	Date:
Mileage:	Mileage:	Mileage:	Mileage:	Mileage:	Mileage:	Mileage:

Week 2

Date:	Date:	Date:	Date:	Date:	Date:	Date:
Mileage:	Mileage:	Mileage:	Mileage:	Mileage:	Mileage:	Mileage:

Week 3

Date:	Date:	Date:	Date:	Date:	Date:	Date:
Mileage:	Mileage:	Mileage:	Mileage:	Mileage:	Mileage:	Mileage:

Week 4

Date:	Date:	Date:	Date:	Date:	Date:	Date:
Mileage:	Mileage:	Mileage:	Mileage:	Mileage:	Mileage:	Mileage:

Week 5

Date:	Date:	Date:	Date:	Date:	Date:	Date:
Mileage:	Mileage:	Mileage:	Mileage:	Mileage:	Mileage:	Mileage:

Week 6

Date:	Date:	Date:	Date:	Date:	Date:	Date:
Mileage:	Mileage:	Mileage:	Mileage:	Mileage:	Mileage:	Mileage:

Ana/Vo2 CARDIO INTERVALS

(Hvi's) mcw est. '13

Date:	am or pm	Intervals:
W.O.D.:	rps/rnds/lps	HrMx%
1		
2		
3		
4		
5		
6		
7		
8		
9		
10		
11		
12		
	A.L.O.I @:	

Ana/Vo2 CARDIO INTERVALS

(Hvi's) mcw est. '13

Date:	am or pm	Intervals:
W.O.D.:	rps/rnds/lps	HrMx%
1		
2		
3		
4		
5		
6		
7		
8		
9		
10		
11		
12		
	A.L.O.I @:	

Ana/Vo2 CARDIO INTERVALS

(Hvi's) mcw est. '13

Date:	am or pm	Intervals:
W.O.D.:	rps/rnds/lps	HrMx%
1		
2		
3		
4		
5		
6		
7		
8		
9		
10		
11		
12		
	A.L.O.I @:	

Ana/Vo2 CARDIO INTERVALS

(Hvi's) mcw est. '13

Date:	am or pm	Intervals:
W.O.D.:	rps/rnds/lps	HrMx%
1		
2		
3		
4		
5		
6		
7		
8		
9		
10		
11		
12		
	A.L.O.I @:	

Ana/Vo2 CARDIO INTERVALS

(Hvi's) mcw est. '13

Date:	am or pm	Intervals:
W.O.D.:	rps/rnds/lps	HrMx%
1		
2		
3		
4		
5		
6		
7		
8		
9		
10		
11		
12		
	A.L.O.I @:	

Ana/Vo2 CARDIO INTERVALS

(Hvi's) mcw est. '13

Date:	am or pm	Intervals:
W.O.D.:	rps/rnds/lps	HrMx%
1		
2		
3		
4		
5		
6		
7		
8		
9		
10		
11		
12		
	A.L.O.I @:	

Ana/Vo2 CARDIO INTERVALS

(Hvi's) mcw est. '13

	Date:	am or pm	Intervals:
	W.O.D.:	rps/rnds/lps	HrMx%
1			
2			
3			
4			
5			
6			
7			
8			
9			
10			
11			
12			
		A.L.O.I @:	

Ana/Vo2 CARDIO INTERVALS

(Hvi's) mcw est. '13

	Date:	am or pm	Intervals:
	W.O.D.:	rps/rnds/lps	HrMx%
1			
2			
3			
4			
5			
6			
7			
8			
9			
10			
11			
12			
		A.L.O.I @:	

Ana/Vo2 CARDIO INTERVALS

(Hvi's) mcw est. '13

	Date:	am or pm	Intervals:
	W.O.D.:	rps/rnds/lps	HrMx%
1			
2			
3			
4			
5			
6			
7			
8			
9			
10			
11			
12			
		A.L.O.I @:	

Ana/Vo2 CARDIO INTERVALS

(Hvi's) mcw est. '13

	Date:	am or pm	Intervals:
	W.O.D.:	rps/rnds/lps	HrMx%
1			
2			
3			
4			
5			
6			
7			
8			
9			
10			
11			
12			
		A.L.O.I @:	

Ana/Vo2 CARDIO INTERVALS

(Hvi's) mcw est. '13

	Date:	am or pm	Intervals:
	W.O.D.:	rps/rnds/lps	HrMx%
1			
2			
3			
4			
5			
6			
7			
8			
9			
10			
11			
12			
		A.L.O.I @:	

Ana/Vo2 CARDIO INTERVALS

(Hvi's) mcw est. '13

	Date:	am or pm	Intervals:
	W.O.D.:	rps/rnds/lps	HrMx%
1			
2			
3			
4			
5			
6			
7			
8			
9			
10			
11			
12			
		A.L.O.I @:	

Ana/Vo2 CARDIO INTERVALS
(Hvi's) mcw est. '13

	Date:	am or pm	Intervals:
	W.O.D.:	rps/rnds/lps	HrMx%
1			
2			
3			
4			
5			
6			
7			
8			
9			
10			
11			
12			
		A.L.O.I @:	

Ana/Vo2 CARDIO INTERVALS
(Hvi's) mcw est. '13

	Date:	am or pm	Intervals:
	W.O.D.:	rps/rnds/lps	HrMx%
1			
2			
3			
4			
5			
6			
7			
8			
9			
10			
11			
12			
		A.L.O.I @:	

Ana/Vo2 CARDIO INTERVALS
(Hvi's) mcw est. '13

	Date:	am or pm	Intervals:
	W.O.D.:	rps/rnds/lps	HrMx%
1			
2			
3			
4			
5			
6			
7			
8			
9			
10			
11			
12			
		A.L.O.I @:	

Ana/Vo2 CARDIO INTERVALS
(Hvi's) mcw est. '13

	Date:	am or pm	Intervals:
	W.O.D.:	rps/rnds/lps	HrMx%
1			
2			
3			
4			
5			
6			
7			
8			
9			
10			
11			
12			
		A.L.O.I @:	

Ana/Vo2 CARDIO INTERVALS
(Hvi's) mcw est. '13

	Date:	am or pm	Intervals:
	W.O.D.:	rps/rnds/lps	HrMx%
1			
2			
3			
4			
5			
6			
7			
8			
9			
10			
11			
12			
		A.L.O.I @:	

Ana/Vo2 CARDIO INTERVALS
(Hvi's) mcw est. '13

	Date:	am or pm	Intervals:
	W.O.D.:	rps/rnds/lps	HrMx%
1			
2			
3			
4			
5			
6			
7			
8			
9			
10			
11			
12			
		A.L.O.I @:	

Ana/Vo2 CARDIO INTERVALS
(Hvi's) mcw est. '13

	Date:	am or pm	Intervals:
	W.O.D.:	rps/rnds/lps	HrMx%
1			
2			
3			
4			
5			
6			
7			
8			
9			
10			
11			
12			
		A.L.O.I @:	

Ana/Vo2 CARDIO INTERVALS
(Hvi's) mcw est. '13

	Date:	am or pm	Intervals:
	W.O.D.:	rps/rnds/lps	HrMx%
1			
2			
3			
4			
5			
6			
7			
8			
9			
10			
11			
12			
		A.L.O.I @:	

Ana/Vo2 CARDIO INTERVALS
(Hvi's) mcw est. '13

	Date:	am or pm	Intervals:
	W.O.D.:	rps/rnds/lps	HrMx%
1			
2			
3			
4			
5			
6			
7			
8			
9			
10			
11			
12			
		A.L.O.I @:	

Ana/Vo2 CARDIO INTERVALS
(Hvi's) mcw est. '13

	Date:	am or pm	Intervals:
	W.O.D.:	rps/rnds/lps	HrMx%
1			
2			
3			
4			
5			
6			
7			
8			
9			
10			
11			
12			
		A.L.O.I @:	

Ana/Vo2 CARDIO INTERVALS
(Hvi's) mcw est. '13

	Date:	am or pm	Intervals:
	W.O.D.:	rps/rnds/lps	HrMx%
1			
2			
3			
4			
5			
6			
7			
8			
9			
10			
11			
12			
		A.L.O.I @:	

Ana/Vo2 CARDIO INTERVALS
(Hvi's) mcw est. '13

	Date:	am or pm	Intervals:
	W.O.D.:	rps/rnds/lps	HrMx%
1			
2			
3			
4			
5			
6			
7			
8			
9			
10			
11			
12			
		A.L.O.I @:	

Ana/Vo2 CARDIO INTERVALS

(Hvi's) mcw est. '13

	Date:	am or pm	Intervals:
	W.O.D.:	rps/rnds/lps	HrMx%
1			
2			
3			
4			
5			
6			
7			
8			
9			
10			
11			
12			
		A.L.O.I @:	

Ana/Vo2 CARDIO INTERVALS

(Hvi's) mcw est. '13

	Date:	am or pm	Intervals:
	W.O.D.:	rps/rnds/lps	HrMx%
1			
2			
3			
4			
5			
6			
7			
8			
9			
10			
11			
12			
		A.L.O.I @:	

Ana/Vo2 CARDIO INTERVALS

(Hvi's) mcw est. '13

	Date:	am or pm	Intervals:
	W.O.D.:	rps/rnds/lps	HrMx%
1			
2			
3			
4			
5			
6			
7			
8			
9			
10			
11			
12			
		A.L.O.I @:	

Ana/Vo2 CARDIO INTERVALS

(Hvi's) mcw est. '13

	Date:	am or pm	Intervals:
	W.O.D.:	rps/rnds/lps	HrMx%
1			
2			
3			
4			
5			
6			
7			
8			
9			
10			
11			
12			
		A.L.O.I @:	

Ana/Vo2 CARDIO INTERVALS

(Hvi's) mcw est. '13

	Date:	am or pm	Intervals:
	W.O.D.:	rps/rnds/lps	HrMx%
1			
2			
3			
4			
5			
6			
7			
8			
9			
10			
11			
12			
		A.L.O.I @:	

Ana/Vo2 CARDIO INTERVALS

(Hvi's) mcw est. '13

	Date:	am or pm	Intervals:
	W.O.D.:	rps/rnds/lps	HrMx%
1			
2			
3			
4			
5			
6			
7			
8			
9			
10			
11			
12			
		A.L.O.I @:	

FITNESS EVOLUTION NOTES:

Track your Training Effort Intensity Level Zones, Calorie Expense, and Personal Benchmark Record Data

DATE:________ DATA:	DATE:________ DATA:
DATE:________ DATA:	DATE:________ DATA:
DATE:________ DATA:	DATE:________ DATA:
DATE:________ DATA:	DATE:________ DATA:
DATE:________ DATA:	DATE:________ DATA:
DATE:________ DATA:	DATE:________ DATA:
DATE:________ DATA:	DATE:________ DATA:

FITNESS EVOLUTION NOTES:

Track your Training Effort Intensity Level Zones, Calorie Expense, and Personal Benchmark Record Data

DATE:__________ DATA:	DATE:__________ DATA:
DATE:__________ DATA:	DATE:__________ DATA:
DATE:__________ DATA:	DATE:__________ DATA:
DATE:__________ DATA:	DATE:__________ DATA:
DATE:__________ DATA:	DATE:__________ DATA:
DATE:__________ DATA:	DATE:__________ DATA:
DATE:__________ DATA:	DATE:__________ DATA:

NOTES:

NOTES:

6 Week Training Calendar
Month Year

SUNDAY	MONDAY	TUESDAY	WEDNESDAY	THURSDAY	FRIDAY	SATURDAY

Week 1

Date:	Date:	Date:	Date:	Date:	Date:	Date:
Mileage:	Mileage:	Mileage:	Mileage:	Mileage:	Mileage:	Mileage:

Week 2

Date:	Date:	Date:	Date:	Date:	Date:	Date:
Mileage:	Mileage:	Mileage:	Mileage:	Mileage:	Mileage:	Mileage:

Week 3

Date:	Date:	Date:	Date:	Date:	Date:	Date:
Mileage:	Mileage:	Mileage:	Mileage:	Mileage:	Mileage:	Mileage:

Week 4

Date:	Date:	Date:	Date:	Date:	Date:	Date:
Mileage:	Mileage:	Mileage:	Mileage:	Mileage:	Mileage:	Mileage:

Week 5

Date:	Date:	Date:	Date:	Date:	Date:	Date:
Mileage:	Mileage:	Mileage:	Mileage:	Mileage:	Mileage:	Mileage:

Week 6

Date:	Date:	Date:	Date:	Date:	Date:	Date:
Mileage:	Mileage:	Mileage:	Mileage:	Mileage:	Mileage:	Mileage:

Ana/Vo2 CARDIO INTERVALS
(Hvi's) mcw est. '13

	Date:	am or pm	Intervals:
	W.O.D.:	rps/rnds/lps	HrMx%
1			
2			
3			
4			
5			
6			
7			
8			
9			
10			
11			
12			
		A.L.O.I @:	

Ana/Vo2 CARDIO INTERVALS
(Hvi's) mcw est. '13

	Date:	am or pm	Intervals:
	W.O.D.:	rps/rnds/lps	HrMx%
1			
2			
3			
4			
5			
6			
7			
8			
9			
10			
11			
12			
		A.L.O.I @:	

Ana/Vo2 CARDIO INTERVALS
(Hvi's) mcw est. '13

	Date:	am or pm	Intervals:
	W.O.D.:	rps/rnds/lps	HrMx%
1			
2			
3			
4			
5			
6			
7			
8			
9			
10			
11			
12			
		A.L.O.I @:	

Ana/Vo2 CARDIO INTERVALS
(Hvi's) mcw est. '13

	Date:	am or pm	Intervals:
	W.O.D.:	rps/rnds/lps	HrMx%
1			
2			
3			
4			
5			
6			
7			
8			
9			
10			
11			
12			
		A.L.O.I @:	

Ana/Vo2 CARDIO INTERVALS
(Hvi's) mcw est. '13

	Date:	am or pm	Intervals:
	W.O.D.:	rps/rnds/lps	HrMx%
1			
2			
3			
4			
5			
6			
7			
8			
9			
10			
11			
12			
		A.L.O.I @:	

Ana/Vo2 CARDIO INTERVALS
(Hvi's) mcw est. '13

	Date:	am or pm	Intervals:
	W.O.D.:	rps/rnds/lps	HrMx%
1			
2			
3			
4			
5			
6			
7			
8			
9			
10			
11			
12			
		A.L.O.I @:	

Ana/Vo2 CARDIO INTERVALS
(Hvi's) mcw est. '13

	Date:	am or pm	Intervals:
	W.O.D.:	rps/rnds/lps	HrMx%
1			
2			
3			
4			
5			
6			
7			
8			
9			
10			
11			
12			
		A.L.O.I @:	

Ana/Vo2 CARDIO INTERVALS
(Hvi's) mcw est. '13

	Date:	am or pm	Intervals:
	W.O.D.:	rps/rnds/lps	HrMx%
1			
2			
3			
4			
5			
6			
7			
8			
9			
10			
11			
12			
		A.L.O.I @:	

Ana/Vo2 CARDIO INTERVALS
(Hvi's) mcw est. '13

	Date:	am or pm	Intervals:
	W.O.D.:	rps/rnds/lps	HrMx%
1			
2			
3			
4			
5			
6			
7			
8			
9			
10			
11			
12			
		A.L.O.I @:	

Ana/Vo2 CARDIO INTERVALS
(Hvi's) mcw est. '13

	Date:	am or pm	Intervals:
	W.O.D.:	rps/rnds/lps	HrMx%
1			
2			
3			
4			
5			
6			
7			
8			
9			
10			
11			
12			
		A.L.O.I @:	

Ana/Vo2 CARDIO INTERVALS
(Hvi's) mcw est. '13

	Date:	am or pm	Intervals:
	W.O.D.:	rps/rnds/lps	HrMx%
1			
2			
3			
4			
5			
6			
7			
8			
9			
10			
11			
12			
		A.L.O.I @:	

Ana/Vo2 CARDIO INTERVALS
(Hvi's) mcw est. '13

	Date:	am or pm	Intervals:
	W.O.D.:	rps/rnds/lps	HrMx%
1			
2			
3			
4			
5			
6			
7			
8			
9			
10			
11			
12			
		A.L.O.I @:	

Ana/Vo2 CARDIO INTERVALS
(Hvi's) mcw est. '13

	Date:	am or pm	Intervals:
	W.O.D.:	rps/rnds/lps	HrMx%
1			
2			
3			
4			
5			
6			
7			
8			
9			
10			
11			
12			
		A.L.O.I @:	

Ana/Vo2 CARDIO INTERVALS
(Hvi's) mcw est. '13

	Date:	am or pm	Intervals:
	W.O.D.:	rps/rnds/lps	HrMx%
1			
2			
3			
4			
5			
6			
7			
8			
9			
10			
11			
12			
		A.L.O.I @:	

Ana/Vo2 CARDIO INTERVALS
(Hvi's) mcw est. '13

	Date:	am or pm	Intervals:
	W.O.D.:	rps/rnds/lps	HrMx%
1			
2			
3			
4			
5			
6			
7			
8			
9			
10			
11			
12			
		A.L.O.I @:	

Ana/Vo2 CARDIO INTERVALS
(Hvi's) mcw est. '13

	Date:	am or pm	Intervals:
	W.O.D.:	rps/rnds/lps	HrMx%
1			
2			
3			
4			
5			
6			
7			
8			
9			
10			
11			
12			
		A.L.O.I @:	

Ana/Vo2 CARDIO INTERVALS
(Hvi's) mcw est. '13

	Date:	am or pm	Intervals:
	W.O.D.:	rps/rnds/lps	HrMx%
1			
2			
3			
4			
5			
6			
7			
8			
9			
10			
11			
12			
		A.L.O.I @:	

Ana/Vo2 CARDIO INTERVALS
(Hvi's) mcw est. '13

	Date:	am or pm	Intervals:
	W.O.D.:	rps/rnds/lps	HrMx%
1			
2			
3			
4			
5			
6			
7			
8			
9			
10			
11			
12			
		A.L.O.I @:	

Ana/Vo2 CARDIO INTERVALS
(Hvi's) mcw est. '13

	Date:	am or pm	Intervals:
	W.O.D.:	rps/rnds/lps	HrMx%
1			
2			
3			
4			
5			
6			
7			
8			
9			
10			
11			
12			
		A.L.O.I @:	

Ana/Vo2 CARDIO INTERVALS
(Hvi's) mcw est. '13

	Date:	am or pm	Intervals:
	W.O.D.:	rps/rnds/lps	HrMx%
1			
2			
3			
4			
5			
6			
7			
8			
9			
10			
11			
12			
		A.L.O.I @:	

Ana/Vo2 CARDIO INTERVALS
(Hvi's) mcw est. '13

	Date:	am or pm	Intervals:
	W.O.D.:	rps/rnds/lps	HrMx%
1			
2			
3			
4			
5			
6			
7			
8			
9			
10			
11			
12			
		A.L.O.I @:	

Ana/Vo2 CARDIO INTERVALS
(Hvi's) mcw est. '13

	Date:	am or pm	Intervals:
	W.O.D.:	rps/rnds/lps	HrMx%
1			
2			
3			
4			
5			
6			
7			
8			
9			
10			
11			
12			
		A.L.O.I @:	

Ana/Vo2 CARDIO INTERVALS
(Hvi's) mcw est. '13

	Date:	am or pm	Intervals:
	W.O.D.:	rps/rnds/lps	HrMx%
1			
2			
3			
4			
5			
6			
7			
8			
9			
10			
11			
12			
		A.L.O.I @:	

Ana/Vo2 CARDIO INTERVALS
(Hvi's) mcw est. '13

	Date:	am or pm	Intervals:
	W.O.D.:	rps/rnds/lps	HrMx%
1			
2			
3			
4			
5			
6			
7			
8			
9			
10			
11			
12			
		A.L.O.I @:	

Ana/Vo2 CARDIO INTERVALS

(Hvi's) mcw est. '13

Date:	am or pm	Intervals:
W.O.D.:	rps/rnds/lps	HrMx%
1		
2		
3		
4		
5		
6		
7		
8		
9		
10		
11		
12		
	A.L.O.I @:	

Ana/Vo2 CARDIO INTERVALS

(Hvi's) mcw est. '13

Date:	am or pm	Intervals:
W.O.D.:	rps/rnds/lps	HrMx%
1		
2		
3		
4		
5		
6		
7		
8		
9		
10		
11		
12		
	A.L.O.I @:	

Ana/Vo2 CARDIO INTERVALS

(Hvi's) mcw est. '13

Date:	am or pm	Intervals:
W.O.D.:	rps/rnds/lps	HrMx%
1		
2		
3		
4		
5		
6		
7		
8		
9		
10		
11		
12		
	A.L.O.I @:	

Ana/Vo2 CARDIO INTERVALS

(Hvi's) mcw est. '13

Date:	am or pm	Intervals:
W.O.D.:	rps/rnds/lps	HrMx%
1		
2		
3		
4		
5		
6		
7		
8		
9		
10		
11		
12		
	A.L.O.I @:	

Ana/Vo2 CARDIO INTERVALS

(Hvi's) mcw est. '13

Date:	am or pm	Intervals:
W.O.D.:	rps/rnds/lps	HrMx%
1		
2		
3		
4		
5		
6		
7		
8		
9		
10		
11		
12		
	A.L.O.I @:	

Ana/Vo2 CARDIO INTERVALS

(Hvi's) mcw est. '13

Date:	am or pm	Intervals:
W.O.D.:	rps/rnds/lps	HrMx%
1		
2		
3		
4		
5		
6		
7		
8		
9		
10		
11		
12		
	A.L.O.I @:	

FITNESS EVOLUTION NOTES:

Track your Training Effort Intensity Level Zones, Calorie Expense, and Personal Benchmark Record Data

DATE:__________
DATA:

DATE:__________
DATA:

DATE:__________
DATA:

DATE:__________
DATA:

DATE:__________
DATA:

DATE:__________
DATA:

DATE:__________
DATA:

DATE:__________
DATA:

DATE:__________
DATA:

DATE:__________
DATA:

DATE:__________
DATA:

DATE:__________
DATA:

DATE:__________
DATA:

DATE:__________
DATA:

FITNESS EVOLUTION NOTES:

Track your Training Effort Intensity Level Zones, Calorie Expense, and Personal Benchmark Record Data

DATE:__________ DATA:	DATE:__________ DATA:
DATE:__________ DATA:	DATE:__________ DATA:
DATE:__________ DATA:	DATE:__________ DATA:
DATE:__________ DATA:	DATE:__________ DATA:
DATE:__________ DATA:	DATE:__________ DATA:
DATE:__________ DATA:	DATE:__________ DATA:
DATE:__________ DATA:	DATE:__________ DATA:

NOTES:

NOTES:

6 Week Training Calendar
Month Year

SUNDAY	MONDAY	TUESDAY	WEDNESDAY	THURSDAY	FRIDAY	SATURDAY

Week 1

Date:	Date:	Date:	Date:	Date:	Date:	Date:
Mileage:	Mileage:	Mileage:	Mileage:	Mileage:	Mileage:	Mileage:

Week 2

Date:	Date:	Date:	Date:	Date:	Date:	Date:
Mileage:	Mileage:	Mileage:	Mileage:	Mileage:	Mileage:	Mileage:

Week 3

Date:	Date:	Date:	Date:	Date:	Date:	Date:
Mileage:	Mileage:	Mileage:	Mileage:	Mileage:	Mileage:	Mileage:

Week 4

Date:	Date:	Date:	Date:	Date:	Date:	Date:
Mileage:	Mileage:	Mileage:	Mileage:	Mileage:	Mileage:	Mileage:

Week 5

Date:	Date:	Date:	Date:	Date:	Date:	Date:
Mileage:	Mileage:	Mileage:	Mileage:	Mileage:	Mileage:	Mileage:

Week 6

Date:	Date:	Date:	Date:	Date:	Date:	Date:
Mileage:	Mileage:	Mileage:	Mileage:	Mileage:	Mileage:	Mileage:

Ana/Vo2 CARDIO INTERVALS
(Hvi's) mcw est. '13

	Date:	am or pm	Intervals:
	W.O.D.:	rps/rnds/lps	HrMx%
1			
2			
3			
4			
5			
6			
7			
8			
9			
10			
11			
12			
		A.L.O.I @:	

Ana/Vo2 CARDIO INTERVALS
(Hvi's) mcw est. '13

	Date:	am or pm	Intervals:
	W.O.D.:	rps/rnds/lps	HrMx%
1			
2			
3			
4			
5			
6			
7			
8			
9			
10			
11			
12			
		A.L.O.I @:	

Ana/Vo2 CARDIO INTERVALS
(Hvi's) mcw est. '13

	Date:	am or pm	Intervals:
	W.O.D.:	rps/rnds/lps	HrMx%
1			
2			
3			
4			
5			
6			
7			
8			
9			
10			
11			
12			
		A.L.O.I @:	

Ana/Vo2 CARDIO INTERVALS
(Hvi's) mcw est. '13

	Date:	am or pm	Intervals:
	W.O.D.:	rps/rnds/lps	HrMx%
1			
2			
3			
4			
5			
6			
7			
8			
9			
10			
11			
12			
		A.L.O.I @:	

Ana/Vo2 CARDIO INTERVALS
(Hvi's) mcw est. '13

	Date:	am or pm	Intervals:
	W.O.D.:	rps/rnds/lps	HrMx%
1			
2			
3			
4			
5			
6			
7			
8			
9			
10			
11			
12			
		A.L.O.I @:	

Ana/Vo2 CARDIO INTERVALS
(Hvi's) mcw est. '13

	Date:	am or pm	Intervals:
	W.O.D.:	rps/rnds/lps	HrMx%
1			
2			
3			
4			
5			
6			
7			
8			
9			
10			
11			
12			
		A.L.O.I @:	

Ana/Vo2 CARDIO INTERVALS
(Hvi's) mcw est. '13

	Date:	am or pm	Intervals:
	W.O.D.:	rps/rnds/lps	HrMx%
1			
2			
3			
4			
5			
6			
7			
8			
9			
10			
11			
12			
		A.L.O.I @:	

Ana/Vo2 CARDIO INTERVALS
(Hvi's) mcw est. '13

	Date:	am or pm	Intervals:
	W.O.D.:	rps/rnds/lps	HrMx%
1			
2			
3			
4			
5			
6			
7			
8			
9			
10			
11			
12			
		A.L.O.I @:	

Ana/Vo2 CARDIO INTERVALS
(Hvi's) mcw est. '13

	Date:	am or pm	Intervals:
	W.O.D.:	rps/rnds/lps	HrMx%
1			
2			
3			
4			
5			
6			
7			
8			
9			
10			
11			
12			
		A.L.O.I @:	

Ana/Vo2 CARDIO INTERVALS
(Hvi's) mcw est. '13

	Date:	am or pm	Intervals:
	W.O.D.:	rps/rnds/lps	HrMx%
1			
2			
3			
4			
5			
6			
7			
8			
9			
10			
11			
12			
		A.L.O.I @:	

Ana/Vo2 CARDIO INTERVALS
(Hvi's) mcw est. '13

	Date:	am or pm	Intervals:
	W.O.D.:	rps/rnds/lps	HrMx%
1			
2			
3			
4			
5			
6			
7			
8			
9			
10			
11			
12			
		A.L.O.I @:	

Ana/Vo2 CARDIO INTERVALS
(Hvi's) mcw est. '13

	Date:	am or pm	Intervals:
	W.O.D.:	rps/rnds/lps	HrMx%
1			
2			
3			
4			
5			
6			
7			
8			
9			
10			
11			
12			
		A.L.O.I @:	

Ana/Vo2 CARDIO INTERVALS

(Hvi's) mcw est. '13

	Date:	am or pm	Intervals:
	W.O.D.:	rps/rnds/lps	HrMx%
1			
2			
3			
4			
5			
6			
7			
8			
9			
10			
11			
12			
		A.L.O.I @:	

Ana/Vo2 CARDIO INTERVALS

(Hvi's) mcw est. '13

	Date:	am or pm	Intervals:
	W.O.D.:	rps/rnds/lps	HrMx%
1			
2			
3			
4			
5			
6			
7			
8			
9			
10			
11			
12			
		A.L.O.I @:	

Ana/Vo2 CARDIO INTERVALS

(Hvi's) mcw est. '13

	Date:	am or pm	Intervals:
	W.O.D.:	rps/rnds/lps	HrMx%
1			
2			
3			
4			
5			
6			
7			
8			
9			
10			
11			
12			
		A.L.O.I @:	

Ana/Vo2 CARDIO INTERVALS

(Hvi's) mcw est. '13

	Date:	am or pm	Intervals:
	W.O.D.:	rps/rnds/lps	HrMx%
1			
2			
3			
4			
5			
6			
7			
8			
9			
10			
11			
12			
		A.L.O.I @:	

Ana/Vo2 CARDIO INTERVALS

(Hvi's) mcw est. '13

	Date:	am or pm	Intervals:
	W.O.D.:	rps/rnds/lps	HrMx%
1			
2			
3			
4			
5			
6			
7			
8			
9			
10			
11			
12			
		A.L.O.I @:	

Ana/Vo2 CARDIO INTERVALS

(Hvi's) mcw est. '13

	Date:	am or pm	Intervals:
	W.O.D.:	rps/rnds/lps	HrMx%
1			
2			
3			
4			
5			
6			
7			
8			
9			
10			
11			
12			
		A.L.O.I @:	

Ana/Vo2 CARDIO INTERVALS

(Hvi's) mcw est. '13

	Date:	am or pm	Intervals:
	W.O.D.:	rps/rnds/lps	HrMx%
1			
2			
3			
4			
5			
6			
7			
8			
9			
10			
11			
12			
		A.L.O.I @:	

Ana/Vo2 CARDIO INTERVALS

(Hvi's) mcw est. '13

	Date:	am or pm	Intervals:
	W.O.D.:	rps/rnds/lps	HrMx%
1			
2			
3			
4			
5			
6			
7			
8			
9			
10			
11			
12			
		A.L.O.I @:	

Ana/Vo2 CARDIO INTERVALS

(Hvi's) mcw est. '13

	Date:	am or pm	Intervals:
	W.O.D.:	rps/rnds/lps	HrMx%
1			
2			
3			
4			
5			
6			
7			
8			
9			
10			
11			
12			
		A.L.O.I @:	

Ana/Vo2 CARDIO INTERVALS

(Hvi's) mcw est. '13

	Date:	am or pm	Intervals:
	W.O.D.:	rps/rnds/lps	HrMx%
1			
2			
3			
4			
5			
6			
7			
8			
9			
10			
11			
12			
		A.L.O.I @:	

Ana/Vo2 CARDIO INTERVALS

(Hvi's) mcw est. '13

	Date:	am or pm	Intervals:
	W.O.D.:	rps/rnds/lps	HrMx%
1			
2			
3			
4			
5			
6			
7			
8			
9			
10			
11			
12			
		A.L.O.I @:	

Ana/Vo2 CARDIO INTERVALS

(Hvi's) mcw est. '13

	Date:	am or pm	Intervals:
	W.O.D.:	rps/rnds/lps	HrMx%
1			
2			
3			
4			
5			
6			
7			
8			
9			
10			
11			
12			
		A.L.O.I @:	

Ana/Vo2 CARDIO INTERVALS
(Hvi's) mcw est. '13

	Date:	am or pm	Intervals:
	W.O.D.:	rps/rnds/lps	HrMx%
1			
2			
3			
4			
5			
6			
7			
8			
9			
10			
11			
12			
		A.L.O.I @:	

Ana/Vo2 CARDIO INTERVALS
(Hvi's) mcw est. '13

	Date:	am or pm	Intervals:
	W.O.D.:	rps/rnds/lps	HrMx%
1			
2			
3			
4			
5			
6			
7			
8			
9			
10			
11			
12			
		A.L.O.I @:	

Ana/Vo2 CARDIO INTERVALS
(Hvi's) mcw est. '13

	Date:	am or pm	Intervals:
	W.O.D.:	rps/rnds/lps	HrMx%
1			
2			
3			
4			
5			
6			
7			
8			
9			
10			
11			
12			
		A.L.O.I @:	

Ana/Vo2 CARDIO INTERVALS
(Hvi's) mcw est. '13

	Date:	am or pm	Intervals:
	W.O.D.:	rps/rnds/lps	HrMx%
1			
2			
3			
4			
5			
6			
7			
8			
9			
10			
11			
12			
		A.L.O.I @:	

Ana/Vo2 CARDIO INTERVALS
(Hvi's) mcw est. '13

	Date:	am or pm	Intervals:
	W.O.D.:	rps/rnds/lps	HrMx%
1			
2			
3			
4			
5			
6			
7			
8			
9			
10			
11			
12			
		A.L.O.I @:	

Ana/Vo2 CARDIO INTERVALS
(Hvi's) mcw est. '13

	Date:	am or pm	Intervals:
	W.O.D.:	rps/rnds/lps	HrMx%
1			
2			
3			
4			
5			
6			
7			
8			
9			
10			
11			
12			
		A.L.O.I @:	

FITNESS EVOLUTION NOTES:

Track your Training Effort Intensity Level Zones, Calorie Expense, and Personal Benchmark Record Data

DATE: DATA:	DATE: DATA:
DATE: DATA:	DATE: DATA:
DATE: DATA:	DATE: DATA:
DATE: DATA:	DATE: DATA:
DATE: DATA:	DATE: DATA:
DATE: DATA:	DATE: DATA:
DATE: DATA:	DATE: DATA:

FITNESS EVOLUTION NOTES:

Track your Training Effort Intensity Level Zones, Calorie Expense, and Personal Benchmark Record Data

DATE:______ DATA:	DATE:______ DATA:
DATE:______ DATA:	DATE:______ DATA:
DATE:______ DATA:	DATE:______ DATA:
DATE:______ DATA:	DATE:______ DATA:
DATE:______ DATA:	DATE:______ DATA:
DATE:______ DATA:	DATE:______ DATA:
DATE:______ DATA:	DATE:______ DATA:

NOTES:

NOTES:

6 Week Training Calendar
Month Year

SUNDAY	MONDAY	TUESDAY	WEDNESDAY	THURSDAY	FRIDAY	SATURDAY
Week 1						
Date:	Date:	Date:	Date:	Date:	Date:	Date:
Mileage:	Mileage:	Mileage:	Mileage:	Mileage:	Mileage:	Mileage:
Week 2						
Date:	Date:	Date:	Date:	Date:	Date:	Date:
Mileage:	Mileage:	Mileage:	Mileage:	Mileage:	Mileage:	Mileage:
Week 3						
Date:	Date:	Date:	Date:	Date:	Date:	Date:
Mileage:	Mileage:	Mileage:	Mileage:	Mileage:	Mileage:	Mileage:
Week 4						
Date:	Date:	Date:	Date:	Date:	Date:	Date:
Mileage:	Mileage:	Mileage:	Mileage:	Mileage:	Mileage:	Mileage:
Week 5						
Date:	Date:	Date:	Date:	Date:	Date:	Date:
Mileage:	Mileage:	Mileage:	Mileage:	Mileage:	Mileage:	Mileage:
Week 6						
Date:	Date:	Date:	Date:	Date:	Date:	Date:
Mileage:	Mileage:	Mileage:	Mileage:	Mileage:	Mileage:	Mileage:

Ana/Vo2 CARDIO INTERVALS

(Hvi's) mcw est. '13

	Date:	am or pm	Intervals:
	W.O.D.:	rps/rnds/lps	HrMx%
1			
2			
3			
4			
5			
6			
7			
8			
9			
10			
11			
12			
		A.L.O.I @:	

Ana/Vo2 CARDIO INTERVALS

(Hvi's) mcw est. '13

	Date:	am or pm	Intervals:
	W.O.D.:	rps/rnds/lps	HrMx%
1			
2			
3			
4			
5			
6			
7			
8			
9			
10			
11			
12			
		A.L.O.I @:	

Ana/Vo2 CARDIO INTERVALS

(Hvi's) mcw est. '13

	Date:	am or pm	Intervals:
	W.O.D.:	rps/rnds/lps	HrMx%
1			
2			
3			
4			
5			
6			
7			
8			
9			
10			
11			
12			
		A.L.O.I @:	

Ana/Vo2 CARDIO INTERVALS

(Hvi's) mcw est. '13

	Date:	am or pm	Intervals:
	W.O.D.:	rps/rnds/lps	HrMx%
1			
2			
3			
4			
5			
6			
7			
8			
9			
10			
11			
12			
		A.L.O.I @:	

Ana/Vo2 CARDIO INTERVALS

(Hvi's) mcw est. '13

	Date:	am or pm	Intervals:
	W.O.D.:	rps/rnds/lps	HrMx%
1			
2			
3			
4			
5			
6			
7			
8			
9			
10			
11			
12			
		A.L.O.I @:	

Ana/Vo2 CARDIO INTERVALS

(Hvi's) mcw est. '13

	Date:	am or pm	Intervals:
	W.O.D.:	rps/rnds/lps	HrMx%
1			
2			
3			
4			
5			
6			
7			
8			
9			
10			
11			
12			
		A.L.O.I @:	

Ana/Vo2 CARDIO INTERVALS
(Hvi's) mcw est. '13

	Date:	am or pm	Intervals:
	W.O.D.:	rps/rnds/lps	HrMx%
1			
2			
3			
4			
5			
6			
7			
8			
9			
10			
11			
12			
		A.L.O.I @:	

Ana/Vo2 CARDIO INTERVALS
(Hvi's) mcw est. '13

	Date:	am or pm	Intervals:
	W.O.D.:	rps/rnds/lps	HrMx%
1			
2			
3			
4			
5			
6			
7			
8			
9			
10			
11			
12			
		A.L.O.I @:	

Ana/Vo2 CARDIO INTERVALS
(Hvi's) mcw est. '13

	Date:	am or pm	Intervals:
	W.O.D.:	rps/rnds/lps	HrMx%
1			
2			
3			
4			
5			
6			
7			
8			
9			
10			
11			
12			
		A.L.O.I @:	

Ana/Vo2 CARDIO INTERVALS
(Hvi's) mcw est. '13

	Date:	am or pm	Intervals:
	W.O.D.:	rps/rnds/lps	HrMx%
1			
2			
3			
4			
5			
6			
7			
8			
9			
10			
11			
12			
		A.L.O.I @:	

Ana/Vo2 CARDIO INTERVALS
(Hvi's) mcw est. '13

	Date:	am or pm	Intervals:
	W.O.D.:	rps/rnds/lps	HrMx%
1			
2			
3			
4			
5			
6			
7			
8			
9			
10			
11			
12			
		A.L.O.I @:	

Ana/Vo2 CARDIO INTERVALS
(Hvi's) mcw est. '13

	Date:	am or pm	Intervals:
	W.O.D.:	rps/rnds/lps	HrMx%
1			
2			
3			
4			
5			
6			
7			
8			
9			
10			
11			
12			
		A.L.O.I @:	

Ana/Vo2 CARDIO INTERVALS
(Hvi's) mcw est. '13

	Date:	am or pm	Intervals:
	W.O.D.:	rps/rnds/lps	HrMx%
1			
2			
3			
4			
5			
6			
7			
8			
9			
10			
11			
12			
		A.L.O.I @:	

Ana/Vo2 CARDIO INTERVALS
(Hvi's) mcw est. '13

	Date:	am or pm	Intervals:
	W.O.D.:	rps/rnds/lps	HrMx%
1			
2			
3			
4			
5			
6			
7			
8			
9			
10			
11			
12			
		A.L.O.I @:	

Ana/Vo2 CARDIO INTERVALS
(Hvi's) mcw est. '13

	Date:	am or pm	Intervals:
	W.O.D.:	rps/rnds/lps	HrMx%
1			
2			
3			
4			
5			
6			
7			
8			
9			
10			
11			
12			
		A.L.O.I @:	

Ana/Vo2 CARDIO INTERVALS
(Hvi's) mcw est. '13

	Date:	am or pm	Intervals:
	W.O.D.:	rps/rnds/lps	HrMx%
1			
2			
3			
4			
5			
6			
7			
8			
9			
10			
11			
12			
		A.L.O.I @:	

Ana/Vo2 CARDIO INTERVALS
(Hvi's) mcw est. '13

	Date:	am or pm	Intervals:
	W.O.D.:	rps/rnds/lps	HrMx%
1			
2			
3			
4			
5			
6			
7			
8			
9			
10			
11			
12			
		A.L.O.I @:	

Ana/Vo2 CARDIO INTERVALS
(Hvi's) mcw est. '13

	Date:	am or pm	Intervals:
	W.O.D.:	rps/rnds/lps	HrMx%
1			
2			
3			
4			
5			
6			
7			
8			
9			
10			
11			
12			
		A.L.O.I @:	

Ana/Vo2 CARDIO INTERVALS
(Hvi's) mcw est. '13

	Date:	am or pm	Intervals:
	W.O.D.:	rps/rnds/lps	HrMx%
1			
2			
3			
4			
5			
6			
7			
8			
9			
10			
11			
12			
		A.L.O.I @:	

Ana/Vo2 CARDIO INTERVALS
(Hvi's) mcw est. '13

	Date:	am or pm	Intervals:
	W.O.D.:	rps/rnds/lps	HrMx%
1			
2			
3			
4			
5			
6			
7			
8			
9			
10			
11			
12			
		A.L.O.I @:	

Ana/Vo2 CARDIO INTERVALS
(Hvi's) mcw est. '13

	Date:	am or pm	Intervals:
	W.O.D.:	rps/rnds/lps	HrMx%
1			
2			
3			
4			
5			
6			
7			
8			
9			
10			
11			
12			
		A.L.O.I @:	

Ana/Vo2 CARDIO INTERVALS
(Hvi's) mcw est. '13

	Date:	am or pm	Intervals:
	W.O.D.:	rps/rnds/lps	HrMx%
1			
2			
3			
4			
5			
6			
7			
8			
9			
10			
11			
12			
		A.L.O.I @:	

Ana/Vo2 CARDIO INTERVALS
(Hvi's) mcw est. '13

	Date:	am or pm	Intervals:
	W.O.D.:	rps/rnds/lps	HrMx%
1			
2			
3			
4			
5			
6			
7			
8			
9			
10			
11			
12			
		A.L.O.I @:	

Ana/Vo2 CARDIO INTERVALS
(Hvi's) mcw est. '13

	Date:	am or pm	Intervals:
	W.O.D.:	rps/rnds/lps	HrMx%
1			
2			
3			
4			
5			
6			
7			
8			
9			
10			
11			
12			
		A.L.O.I @:	

Ana/Vo2 CARDIO INTERVALS

(Hvi's) mcw est. '13

	Date:	am or pm	Intervals:
	W.O.D.:	rps/rnds/lps	HrMx%
1			
2			
3			
4			
5			
6			
7			
8			
9			
10			
11			
12			
		A.L.O.I @:	

Ana/Vo2 CARDIO INTERVALS

(Hvi's) mcw est. '13

	Date:	am or pm	Intervals:
	W.O.D.:	rps/rnds/lps	HrMx%
1			
2			
3			
4			
5			
6			
7			
8			
9			
10			
11			
12			
		A.L.O.I @:	

Ana/Vo2 CARDIO INTERVALS

(Hvi's) mcw est. '13

	Date:	am or pm	Intervals:
	W.O.D.:	rps/rnds/lps	HrMx%
1			
2			
3			
4			
5			
6			
7			
8			
9			
10			
11			
12			
		A.L.O.I @:	

Ana/Vo2 CARDIO INTERVALS

(Hvi's) mcw est. '13

	Date:	am or pm	Intervals:
	W.O.D.:	rps/rnds/lps	HrMx%
1			
2			
3			
4			
5			
6			
7			
8			
9			
10			
11			
12			
		A.L.O.I @:	

Ana/Vo2 CARDIO INTERVALS

(Hvi's) mcw est. '13

	Date:	am or pm	Intervals:
	W.O.D.:	rps/rnds/lps	HrMx%
1			
2			
3			
4			
5			
6			
7			
8			
9			
10			
11			
12			
		A.L.O.I @:	

Ana/Vo2 CARDIO INTERVALS

(Hvi's) mcw est. '13

	Date:	am or pm	Intervals:
	W.O.D.:	rps/rnds/lps	HrMx%
1			
2			
3			
4			
5			
6			
7			
8			
9			
10			
11			
12			
		A.L.O.I @:	

FITNESS EVOLUTION NOTES:

Track your Training Effort Intensity Level Zones, Calorie Expense, and Personal Benchmark Record Data

DATE:__________ DATA:	DATE:__________ DATA:
DATE:__________ DATA:	DATE:__________ DATA:
DATE:__________ DATA:	DATE:__________ DATA:
DATE:__________ DATA:	DATE:__________ DATA:
DATE:__________ DATA:	DATE:__________ DATA:
DATE:__________ DATA:	DATE:__________ DATA:
DATE:__________ DATA:	DATE:__________ DATA:

FITNESS EVOLUTION NOTES:

Track your Training Effort Intensity Level Zones, Calorie Expense, and Personal Benchmark Record Data

DATE:__________ DATA:	DATE:__________ DATA:
DATE:__________ DATA:	DATE:__________ DATA:
DATE:__________ DATA:	DATE:__________ DATA:
DATE:__________ DATA:	DATE:__________ DATA:
DATE:__________ DATA:	DATE:__________ DATA:
DATE:__________ DATA:	DATE:__________ DATA:
DATE:__________ DATA:	DATE:__________ DATA:

NOTES:

NOTES:

6 Week Training Calendar
Month Year

SUNDAY	MONDAY	TUESDAY	WEDNESDAY	THURSDAY	FRIDAY	SATURDAY

Week 1

Date:	Date:	Date:	Date:	Date:	Date:	Date:
Mileage:	Mileage:	Mileage:	Mileage:	Mileage:	Mileage:	Mileage:

Week 2

Date:	Date:	Date:	Date:	Date:	Date:	Date:
Mileage:	Mileage:	Mileage:	Mileage:	Mileage:	Mileage:	Mileage:

Week 3

Date:	Date:	Date:	Date:	Date:	Date:	Date:
Mileage:	Mileage:	Mileage:	Mileage:	Mileage:	Mileage:	Mileage:

Week 4

Date:	Date:	Date:	Date:	Date:	Date:	Date:
Mileage:	Mileage:	Mileage:	Mileage:	Mileage:	Mileage:	Mileage:

Week 5

Date:	Date:	Date:	Date:	Date:	Date:	Date:
Mileage:	Mileage:	Mileage:	Mileage:	Mileage:	Mileage:	Mileage:

Week 6

Date:	Date:	Date:	Date:	Date:	Date:	Date:
Mileage:	Mileage:	Mileage:	Mileage:	Mileage:	Mileage:	Mileage:

Ana/Vo2 CARDIO INTERVALS

(Hvi's) mcw est. '13

	Date:	am or pm	Intervals:
	W.O.D.:	rps/rnds/lps	HrMx%
1			
2			
3			
4			
5			
6			
7			
8			
9			
10			
11			
12			
		A.L.O.I @:	

Ana/Vo2 CARDIO INTERVALS

(Hvi's) mcw est. '13

	Date:	am or pm	Intervals:
	W.O.D.:	rps/rnds/lps	HrMx%
1			
2			
3			
4			
5			
6			
7			
8			
9			
10			
11			
12			
		A.L.O.I @:	

Ana/Vo2 CARDIO INTERVALS

(Hvi's) mcw est. '13

	Date:	am or pm	Intervals:
	W.O.D.:	rps/rnds/lps	HrMx%
1			
2			
3			
4			
5			
6			
7			
8			
9			
10			
11			
12			
		A.L.O.I @:	

Ana/Vo2 CARDIO INTERVALS

(Hvi's) mcw est. '13

	Date:	am or pm	Intervals:
	W.O.D.:	rps/rnds/lps	HrMx%
1			
2			
3			
4			
5			
6			
7			
8			
9			
10			
11			
12			
		A.L.O.I @:	

Ana/Vo2 CARDIO INTERVALS

(Hvi's) mcw est. '13

	Date:	am or pm	Intervals:
	W.O.D.:	rps/rnds/lps	HrMx%
1			
2			
3			
4			
5			
6			
7			
8			
9			
10			
11			
12			
		A.L.O.I @:	

Ana/Vo2 CARDIO INTERVALS

(Hvi's) mcw est. '13

	Date:	am or pm	Intervals:
	W.O.D.:	rps/rnds/lps	HrMx%
1			
2			
3			
4			
5			
6			
7			
8			
9			
10			
11			
12			
		A.L.O.I @:	

Ana/Vo2 CARDIO INTERVALS

(Hvi's) mcw est. '13

	Date:	am or pm	Intervals:
	W.O.D.:	rps/rnds/lps	HrMx%
1			
2			
3			
4			
5			
6			
7			
8			
9			
10			
11			
12			
		A.L.O.I @:	

Ana/Vo2 CARDIO INTERVALS

(Hvi's) mcw est. '13

	Date:	am or pm	Intervals:
	W.O.D.:	rps/rnds/lps	HrMx%
1			
2			
3			
4			
5			
6			
7			
8			
9			
10			
11			
12			
		A.L.O.I @:	

Ana/Vo2 CARDIO INTERVALS

(Hvi's) mcw est. '13

	Date:	am or pm	Intervals:
	W.O.D.:	rps/rnds/lps	HrMx%
1			
2			
3			
4			
5			
6			
7			
8			
9			
10			
11			
12			
		A.L.O.I @:	

Ana/Vo2 CARDIO INTERVALS

(Hvi's) mcw est. '13

	Date:	am or pm	Intervals:
	W.O.D.:	rps/rnds/lps	HrMx%
1			
2			
3			
4			
5			
6			
7			
8			
9			
10			
11			
12			
		A.L.O.I @:	

Ana/Vo2 CARDIO INTERVALS

(Hvi's) mcw est. '13

	Date:	am or pm	Intervals:
	W.O.D.:	rps/rnds/lps	HrMx%
1			
2			
3			
4			
5			
6			
7			
8			
9			
10			
11			
12			
		A.L.O.I @:	

Ana/Vo2 CARDIO INTERVALS

(Hvi's) mcw est. '13

	Date:	am or pm	Intervals:
	W.O.D.:	rps/rnds/lps	HrMx%
1			
2			
3			
4			
5			
6			
7			
8			
9			
10			
11			
12			
		A.L.O.I @:	

Ana/Vo2 CARDIO INTERVALS

(Hvi's) mcw est. '13

	Date:	am or pm	Intervals:
	W.O.D.:	rps/rnds/lps	HrMx%
1			
2			
3			
4			
5			
6			
7			
8			
9			
10			
11			
12			
		A.L.O.I @:	

Ana/Vo2 CARDIO INTERVALS

(Hvi's) mcw est. '13

	Date:	am or pm	Intervals:
	W.O.D.:	rps/rnds/lps	HrMx%
1			
2			
3			
4			
5			
6			
7			
8			
9			
10			
11			
12			
		A.L.O.I @:	

Ana/Vo2 CARDIO INTERVALS

(Hvi's) mcw est. '13

	Date:	am or pm	Intervals:
	W.O.D.:	rps/rnds/lps	HrMx%
1			
2			
3			
4			
5			
6			
7			
8			
9			
10			
11			
12			
		A.L.O.I @:	

Ana/Vo2 CARDIO INTERVALS

(Hvi's) mcw est. '13

	Date:	am or pm	Intervals:
	W.O.D.:	rps/rnds/lps	HrMx%
1			
2			
3			
4			
5			
6			
7			
8			
9			
10			
11			
12			
		A.L.O.I @:	

Ana/Vo2 CARDIO INTERVALS

(Hvi's) mcw est. '13

	Date:	am or pm	Intervals:
	W.O.D.:	rps/rnds/lps	HrMx%
1			
2			
3			
4			
5			
6			
7			
8			
9			
10			
11			
12			
		A.L.O.I @:	

Ana/Vo2 CARDIO INTERVALS

(Hvi's) mcw est. '13

	Date:	am or pm	Intervals:
	W.O.D.:	rps/rnds/lps	HrMx%
1			
2			
3			
4			
5			
6			
7			
8			
9			
10			
11			
12			
		A.L.O.I @:	

Ana/Vo2 CARDIO INTERVALS

(Hvi's) mcw est. '13

	Date:	am or pm	Intervals:
	W.O.D.:	rps/rnds/lps	HrMx%
1			
2			
3			
4			
5			
6			
7			
8			
9			
10			
11			
12			
		A.L.O.I @:	

Ana/Vo2 CARDIO INTERVALS

(Hvi's) mcw est. '13

	Date:	am or pm	Intervals:
	W.O.D.:	rps/rnds/lps	HrMx%
1			
2			
3			
4			
5			
6			
7			
8			
9			
10			
11			
12			
		A.L.O.I @:	

Ana/Vo2 CARDIO INTERVALS

(Hvi's) mcw est. '13

	Date:	am or pm	Intervals:
	W.O.D.:	rps/rnds/lps	HrMx%
1			
2			
3			
4			
5			
6			
7			
8			
9			
10			
11			
12			
		A.L.O.I @:	

Ana/Vo2 CARDIO INTERVALS

(Hvi's) mcw est. '13

	Date:	am or pm	Intervals:
	W.O.D.:	rps/rnds/lps	HrMx%
1			
2			
3			
4			
5			
6			
7			
8			
9			
10			
11			
12			
		A.L.O.I @:	

Ana/Vo2 CARDIO INTERVALS

(Hvi's) mcw est. '13

	Date:	am or pm	Intervals:
	W.O.D.:	rps/rnds/lps	HrMx%
1			
2			
3			
4			
5			
6			
7			
8			
9			
10			
11			
12			
		A.L.O.I @:	

Ana/Vo2 CARDIO INTERVALS

(Hvi's) mcw est. '13

	Date:	am or pm	Intervals:
	W.O.D.:	rps/rnds/lps	HrMx%
1			
2			
3			
4			
5			
6			
7			
8			
9			
10			
11			
12			
		A.L.O.I @:	

Ana/Vo2 CARDIO INTERVALS

(Hvi's) mcw est. '13

	Date:	am or pm	Intervals:
	W.O.D.:	rps/rnds/lps	HrMx%
1			
2			
3			
4			
5			
6			
7			
8			
9			
10			
11			
12			
		A.L.O.I @:	

Ana/Vo2 CARDIO INTERVALS

(Hvi's) mcw est. '13

	Date:	am or pm	Intervals:
	W.O.D.:	rps/rnds/lps	HrMx%
1			
2			
3			
4			
5			
6			
7			
8			
9			
10			
11			
12			
		A.L.O.I @:	

Ana/Vo2 CARDIO INTERVALS

(Hvi's) mcw est. '13

	Date:	am or pm	Intervals:
	W.O.D.:	rps/rnds/lps	HrMx%
1			
2			
3			
4			
5			
6			
7			
8			
9			
10			
11			
12			
		A.L.O.I @:	

Ana/Vo2 CARDIO INTERVALS

(Hvi's) mcw est. '13

	Date:	am or pm	Intervals:
	W.O.D.:	rps/rnds/lps	HrMx%
1			
2			
3			
4			
5			
6			
7			
8			
9			
10			
11			
12			
		A.L.O.I @:	

Ana/Vo2 CARDIO INTERVALS

(Hvi's) mcw est. '13

	Date:	am or pm	Intervals:
	W.O.D.:	rps/rnds/lps	HrMx%
1			
2			
3			
4			
5			
6			
7			
8			
9			
10			
11			
12			
		A.L.O.I @:	

Ana/Vo2 CARDIO INTERVALS

(Hvi's) mcw est. '13

	Date:	am or pm	Intervals:
	W.O.D.:	rps/rnds/lps	HrMx%
1			
2			
3			
4			
5			
6			
7			
8			
9			
10			
11			
12			
		A.L.O.I @:	

FITNESS EVOLUTION NOTES:

Track your Training Effort Intensity Level Zones, Calorie Expense, and Personal Benchmark Record Data

DATE:__________ DATA:	DATE:__________ DATA:
DATE:__________ DATA:	DATE:__________ DATA:
DATE:__________ DATA:	DATE:__________ DATA:
DATE:__________ DATA:	DATE:__________ DATA:
DATE:__________ DATA:	DATE:__________ DATA:
DATE:__________ DATA:	DATE:__________ DATA:
DATE:__________ DATA:	DATE:__________ DATA:

FITNESS EVOLUTION NOTES:

Track your Training Effort Intensity Level Zones, Calorie Expense, and Personal Benchmark Record Data

DATE:__________ DATA:	DATE:__________ DATA:
DATE:__________ DATA:	DATE:__________ DATA:
DATE:__________ DATA:	DATE:__________ DATA:
DATE:__________ DATA:	DATE:__________ DATA:
DATE:__________ DATA:	DATE:__________ DATA:
DATE:__________ DATA:	DATE:__________ DATA:
DATE:__________ DATA:	DATE:__________ DATA:

NOTES:

NOTES:

6 Week Training Calendar

Month Year

SUNDAY	MONDAY	TUESDAY	WEDNESDAY	THURSDAY	FRIDAY	SATURDAY
Week 1						
Date:	Date:	Date:	Date:	Date:	Date:	Date:
Mileage:	Mileage:	Mileage:	Mileage:	Mileage:	Mileage:	Mileage:
Week 2						
Date:	Date:	Date:	Date:	Date:	Date:	Date:
Mileage:	Mileage:	Mileage:	Mileage:	Mileage:	Mileage:	Mileage:
Week 3						
Date:	Date:	Date:	Date:	Date:	Date:	Date:
Mileage:	Mileage:	Mileage:	Mileage:	Mileage:	Mileage:	Mileage:
Week 4						
Date:	Date:	Date:	Date:	Date:	Date:	Date:
Mileage:	Mileage:	Mileage:	Mileage:	Mileage:	Mileage:	Mileage:
Week 5						
Date:	Date:	Date:	Date:	Date:	Date:	Date:
Mileage:	Mileage:	Mileage:	Mileage:	Mileage:	Mileage:	Mileage:
Week 6						
Date:	Date:	Date:	Date:	Date:	Date:	Date:
Mileage:	Mileage:	Mileage:	Mileage:	Mileage:	Mileage:	Mileage:

Ana/Vo2 CARDIO INTERVALS

(Hvi's) mcw est. '13

	Date:	am or pm	Intervals:
	W.O.D.:	rps/rnds/lps	HrMx%
1			
2			
3			
4			
5			
6			
7			
8			
9			
10			
11			
12			
		A.L.O.I @:	

Ana/Vo2 CARDIO INTERVALS

(Hvi's) mcw est. '13

	Date:	am or pm	Intervals:
	W.O.D.:	rps/rnds/lps	HrMx%
1			
2			
3			
4			
5			
6			
7			
8			
9			
10			
11			
12			
		A.L.O.I @:	

Ana/Vo2 CARDIO INTERVALS

(Hvi's) mcw est. '13

	Date:	am or pm	Intervals:
	W.O.D.:	rps/rnds/lps	HrMx%
1			
2			
3			
4			
5			
6			
7			
8			
9			
10			
11			
12			
		A.L.O.I @:	

Ana/Vo2 CARDIO INTERVALS

(Hvi's) mcw est. '13

	Date:	am or pm	Intervals:
	W.O.D.:	rps/rnds/lps	HrMx%
1			
2			
3			
4			
5			
6			
7			
8			
9			
10			
11			
12			
		A.L.O.I @:	

Ana/Vo2 CARDIO INTERVALS

(Hvi's) mcw est. '13

	Date:	am or pm	Intervals:
	W.O.D.:	rps/rnds/lps	HrMx%
1			
2			
3			
4			
5			
6			
7			
8			
9			
10			
11			
12			
		A.L.O.I @:	

Ana/Vo2 CARDIO INTERVALS

(Hvi's) mcw est. '13

	Date:	am or pm	Intervals:
	W.O.D.:	rps/rnds/lps	HrMx%
1			
2			
3			
4			
5			
6			
7			
8			
9			
10			
11			
12			
		A.L.O.I @:	

Ana/Vo2 CARDIO INTERVALS
(Hvi's) mcw est. '13

	Date:	am or pm	Intervals:
	W.O.D.:	rps/rnds/lps	HrMx%
1			
2			
3			
4			
5			
6			
7			
8			
9			
10			
11			
12			
		A.L.O.I @:	

Ana/Vo2 CARDIO INTERVALS
(Hvi's) mcw est. '13

	Date:	am or pm	Intervals:
	W.O.D.:	rps/rnds/lps	HrMx%
1			
2			
3			
4			
5			
6			
7			
8			
9			
10			
11			
12			
		A.L.O.I @:	

Ana/Vo2 CARDIO INTERVALS
(Hvi's) mcw est. '13

	Date:	am or pm	Intervals:
	W.O.D.:	rps/rnds/lps	HrMx%
1			
2			
3			
4			
5			
6			
7			
8			
9			
10			
11			
12			
		A.L.O.I @:	

Ana/Vo2 CARDIO INTERVALS
(Hvi's) mcw est. '13

	Date:	am or pm	Intervals:
	W.O.D.:	rps/rnds/lps	HrMx%
1			
2			
3			
4			
5			
6			
7			
8			
9			
10			
11			
12			
		A.L.O.I @:	

Ana/Vo2 CARDIO INTERVALS
(Hvi's) mcw est. '13

	Date:	am or pm	Intervals:
	W.O.D.:	rps/rnds/lps	HrMx%
1			
2			
3			
4			
5			
6			
7			
8			
9			
10			
11			
12			
		A.L.O.I @:	

Ana/Vo2 CARDIO INTERVALS
(Hvi's) mcw est. '13

	Date:	am or pm	Intervals:
	W.O.D.:	rps/rnds/lps	HrMx%
1			
2			
3			
4			
5			
6			
7			
8			
9			
10			
11			
12			
		A.L.O.I @:	

Ana/Vo2 CARDIO INTERVALS
(Hvi's) mcw est. '13

	Date:	am or pm	Intervals:
	W.O.D.:	rps/rnds/lps	HrMx%
1			
2			
3			
4			
5			
6			
7			
8			
9			
10			
11			
12			
		A.L.O.I @:	

Ana/Vo2 CARDIO INTERVALS
(Hvi's) mcw est. '13

	Date:	am or pm	Intervals:
	W.O.D.:	rps/rnds/lps	HrMx%
1			
2			
3			
4			
5			
6			
7			
8			
9			
10			
11			
12			
		A.L.O.I @:	

Ana/Vo2 CARDIO INTERVALS
(Hvi's) mcw est. '13

	Date:	am or pm	Intervals:
	W.O.D.:	rps/rnds/lps	HrMx%
1			
2			
3			
4			
5			
6			
7			
8			
9			
10			
11			
12			
		A.L.O.I @:	

Ana/Vo2 CARDIO INTERVALS
(Hvi's) mcw est. '13

	Date:	am or pm	Intervals:
	W.O.D.:	rps/rnds/lps	HrMx%
1			
2			
3			
4			
5			
6			
7			
8			
9			
10			
11			
12			
		A.L.O.I @:	

Ana/Vo2 CARDIO INTERVALS
(Hvi's) mcw est. '13

	Date:	am or pm	Intervals:
	W.O.D.:	rps/rnds/lps	HrMx%
1			
2			
3			
4			
5			
6			
7			
8			
9			
10			
11			
12			
		A.L.O.I @:	

Ana/Vo2 CARDIO INTERVALS
(Hvi's) mcw est. '13

	Date:	am or pm	Intervals:
	W.O.D.:	rps/rnds/lps	HrMx%
1			
2			
3			
4			
5			
6			
7			
8			
9			
10			
11			
12			
		A.L.O.I @:	

Ana/Vo2 CARDIO INTERVALS
(Hvi's) mcw est. '13

	Date:	am or pm	Intervals:
	W.O.D.:	rps/rnds/lps	HrMx%
1			
2			
3			
4			
5			
6			
7			
8			
9			
10			
11			
12			
		A.L.O.I @:	

Ana/Vo2 CARDIO INTERVALS
(Hvi's) mcw est. '13

	Date:	am or pm	Intervals:
	W.O.D.:	rps/rnds/lps	HrMx%
1			
2			
3			
4			
5			
6			
7			
8			
9			
10			
11			
12			
		A.L.O.I @:	

Ana/Vo2 CARDIO INTERVALS
(Hvi's) mcw est. '13

	Date:	am or pm	Intervals:
	W.O.D.:	rps/rnds/lps	HrMx%
1			
2			
3			
4			
5			
6			
7			
8			
9			
10			
11			
12			
		A.L.O.I @:	

Ana/Vo2 CARDIO INTERVALS
(Hvi's) mcw est. '13

	Date:	am or pm	Intervals:
	W.O.D.:	rps/rnds/lps	HrMx%
1			
2			
3			
4			
5			
6			
7			
8			
9			
10			
11			
12			
		A.L.O.I @:	

Ana/Vo2 CARDIO INTERVALS
(Hvi's) mcw est. '13

	Date:	am or pm	Intervals:
	W.O.D.:	rps/rnds/lps	HrMx%
1			
2			
3			
4			
5			
6			
7			
8			
9			
10			
11			
12			
		A.L.O.I @:	

Ana/Vo2 CARDIO INTERVALS
(Hvi's) mcw est. '13

	Date:	am or pm	Intervals:
	W.O.D.:	rps/rnds/lps	HrMx%
1			
2			
3			
4			
5			
6			
7			
8			
9			
10			
11			
12			
		A.L.O.I @:	

Ana/Vo2 CARDIO INTERVALS

(Hvi's) mcw est. '13

	Date:	am or pm	Intervals:
	W.O.D.:	rps/rnds/lps	HrMx%
1			
2			
3			
4			
5			
6			
7			
8			
9			
10			
11			
12			
		A.L.O.I @:	

Ana/Vo2 CARDIO INTERVALS

(Hvi's) mcw est. '13

	Date:	am or pm	Intervals:
	W.O.D.:	rps/rnds/lps	HrMx%
1			
2			
3			
4			
5			
6			
7			
8			
9			
10			
11			
12			
		A.L.O.I @:	

Ana/Vo2 CARDIO INTERVALS

(Hvi's) mcw est. '13

	Date:	am or pm	Intervals:
	W.O.D.:	rps/rnds/lps	HrMx%
1			
2			
3			
4			
5			
6			
7			
8			
9			
10			
11			
12			
		A.L.O.I @:	

Ana/Vo2 CARDIO INTERVALS

(Hvi's) mcw est. '13

	Date:	am or pm	Intervals:
	W.O.D.:	rps/rnds/lps	HrMx%
1			
2			
3			
4			
5			
6			
7			
8			
9			
10			
11			
12			
		A.L.O.I @:	

Ana/Vo2 CARDIO INTERVALS

(Hvi's) mcw est. '13

	Date:	am or pm	Intervals:
	W.O.D.:	rps/rnds/lps	HrMx%
1			
2			
3			
4			
5			
6			
7			
8			
9			
10			
11			
12			
		A.L.O.I @:	

Ana/Vo2 CARDIO INTERVALS

(Hvi's) mcw est. '13

	Date:	am or pm	Intervals:
	W.O.D.:	rps/rnds/lps	HrMx%
1			
2			
3			
4			
5			
6			
7			
8			
9			
10			
11			
12			
		A.L.O.I @:	

FITNESS EVOLUTION NOTES:

Track your Training Effort Intensity Level Zones, Calorie Expense, and Personal Benchmark Record Data

DATE:________ DATA:	DATE:________ DATA:
DATE:________ DATA:	DATE:________ DATA:
DATE:________ DATA:	DATE:________ DATA:
DATE:________ DATA:	DATE:________ DATA:
DATE:________ DATA:	DATE:________ DATA:
DATE:________ DATA:	DATE:________ DATA:
DATE:________ DATA:	DATE:________ DATA:

FITNESS EVOLUTION NOTES:

Track your Training Effort Intensity Level Zones, Calorie Expense, and Personal Benchmark Record Data

DATE:__________ DATA:	DATE:__________ DATA:
DATE:__________ DATA:	DATE:__________ DATA:
DATE:__________ DATA:	DATE:__________ DATA:
DATE:__________ DATA:	DATE:__________ DATA:
DATE:__________ DATA:	DATE:__________ DATA:
DATE:__________ DATA:	DATE:__________ DATA:
DATE:__________ DATA:	DATE:__________ DATA:

NOTES:

NOTES:

6 Week Training Calendar

Month Year

SUNDAY	MONDAY	TUESDAY	WEDNESDAY	THURSDAY	FRIDAY	SATURDAY

Week 1

Date:	Date:	Date:	Date:	Date:	Date:	Date:
Mileage:	Mileage:	Mileage:	Mileage:	Mileage:	Mileage:	Mileage:

Week 2

Date:	Date:	Date:	Date:	Date:	Date:	Date:
Mileage:	Mileage:	Mileage:	Mileage:	Mileage:	Mileage:	Mileage:

Week 3

Date:	Date:	Date:	Date:	Date:	Date:	Date:
Mileage:	Mileage:	Mileage:	Mileage:	Mileage:	Mileage:	Mileage:

Week 4

Date:	Date:	Date:	Date:	Date:	Date:	Date:
Mileage:	Mileage:	Mileage:	Mileage:	Mileage:	Mileage:	Mileage:

Week 5

Date:	Date:	Date:	Date:	Date:	Date:	Date:
Mileage:	Mileage:	Mileage:	Mileage:	Mileage:	Mileage:	Mileage:

Week 6

Date:	Date:	Date:	Date:	Date:	Date:	Date:
Mileage:	Mileage:	Mileage:	Mileage:	Mileage:	Mileage:	Mileage:

Ana/Vo2 CARDIO INTERVALS

(Hvi's) mcw est. '13

	Date:	am or pm	Intervals:
	W.O.D.:	rps/rnds/lps	HrMx%
1			
2			
3			
4			
5			
6			
7			
8			
9			
10			
11			
12			
		A.L.O.I @:	

Ana/Vo2 CARDIO INTERVALS

(Hvi's) mcw est. '13

	Date:	am or pm	Intervals:
	W.O.D.:	rps/rnds/lps	HrMx%
1			
2			
3			
4			
5			
6			
7			
8			
9			
10			
11			
12			
		A.L.O.I @:	

Ana/Vo2 CARDIO INTERVALS

(Hvi's) mcw est. '13

	Date:	am or pm	Intervals:
	W.O.D.:	rps/rnds/lps	HrMx%
1			
2			
3			
4			
5			
6			
7			
8			
9			
10			
11			
12			
		A.L.O.I @:	

Ana/Vo2 CARDIO INTERVALS

(Hvi's) mcw est. '13

	Date:	am or pm	Intervals:
	W.O.D.:	rps/rnds/lps	HrMx%
1			
2			
3			
4			
5			
6			
7			
8			
9			
10			
11			
12			
		A.L.O.I @:	

Ana/Vo2 CARDIO INTERVALS

(Hvi's) mcw est. '13

	Date:	am or pm	Intervals:
	W.O.D.:	rps/rnds/lps	HrMx%
1			
2			
3			
4			
5			
6			
7			
8			
9			
10			
11			
12			
		A.L.O.I @:	

Ana/Vo2 CARDIO INTERVALS

(Hvi's) mcw est. '13

	Date:	am or pm	Intervals:
	W.O.D.:	rps/rnds/lps	HrMx%
1			
2			
3			
4			
5			
6			
7			
8			
9			
10			
11			
12			
		A.L.O.I @:	

Ana/Vo2 CARDIO INTERVALS

(Hvi's) mcw est. '13

	Date:	am or pm	Intervals:
	W.O.D.:	rps/rnds/lps	HrMx%
1			
2			
3			
4			
5			
6			
7			
8			
9			
10			
11			
12			
		A.L.O.I @:	

Ana/Vo2 CARDIO INTERVALS

(Hvi's) mcw est. '13

	Date:	am or pm	Intervals:
	W.O.D.:	rps/rnds/lps	HrMx%
1			
2			
3			
4			
5			
6			
7			
8			
9			
10			
11			
12			
		A.L.O.I @:	

Ana/Vo2 CARDIO INTERVALS

(Hvi's) mcw est. '13

	Date:	am or pm	Intervals:
	W.O.D.:	rps/rnds/lps	HrMx%
1			
2			
3			
4			
5			
6			
7			
8			
9			
10			
11			
12			
		A.L.O.I @:	

Ana/Vo2 CARDIO INTERVALS

(Hvi's) mcw est. '13

	Date:	am or pm	Intervals:
	W.O.D.:	rps/rnds/lps	HrMx%
1			
2			
3			
4			
5			
6			
7			
8			
9			
10			
11			
12			
		A.L.O.I @:	

Ana/Vo2 CARDIO INTERVALS

(Hvi's) mcw est. '13

	Date:	am or pm	Intervals:
	W.O.D.:	rps/rnds/lps	HrMx%
1			
2			
3			
4			
5			
6			
7			
8			
9			
10			
11			
12			
		A.L.O.I @:	

Ana/Vo2 CARDIO INTERVALS

(Hvi's) mcw est. '13

	Date:	am or pm	Intervals:
	W.O.D.:	rps/rnds/lps	HrMx%
1			
2			
3			
4			
5			
6			
7			
8			
9			
10			
11			
12			
		A.L.O.I @:	

Ana/Vo2 CARDIO INTERVALS
(Hvi's) mcw est. '13

	Date:	am or pm	Intervals:
	W.O.D.:	rps/rnds/lps	HrMx%
1			
2			
3			
4			
5			
6			
7			
8			
9			
10			
11			
12			
		A.L.O.I @:	

Ana/Vo2 CARDIO INTERVALS
(Hvi's) mcw est. '13

	Date:	am or pm	Intervals:
	W.O.D.:	rps/rnds/lps	HrMx%
1			
2			
3			
4			
5			
6			
7			
8			
9			
10			
11			
12			
		A.L.O.I @:	

Ana/Vo2 CARDIO INTERVALS
(Hvi's) mcw est. '13

	Date:	am or pm	Intervals:
	W.O.D.:	rps/rnds/lps	HrMx%
1			
2			
3			
4			
5			
6			
7			
8			
9			
10			
11			
12			
		A.L.O.I @:	

Ana/Vo2 CARDIO INTERVALS
(Hvi's) mcw est. '13

	Date:	am or pm	Intervals:
	W.O.D.:	rps/rnds/lps	HrMx%
1			
2			
3			
4			
5			
6			
7			
8			
9			
10			
11			
12			
		A.L.O.I @:	

Ana/Vo2 CARDIO INTERVALS
(Hvi's) mcw est. '13

	Date:	am or pm	Intervals:
	W.O.D.:	rps/rnds/lps	HrMx%
1			
2			
3			
4			
5			
6			
7			
8			
9			
10			
11			
12			
		A.L.O.I @:	

Ana/Vo2 CARDIO INTERVALS
(Hvi's) mcw est. '13

	Date:	am or pm	Intervals:
	W.O.D.:	rps/rnds/lps	HrMx%
1			
2			
3			
4			
5			
6			
7			
8			
9			
10			
11			
12			
		A.L.O.I @:	

Ana/Vo2 CARDIO INTERVALS

(Hvi's) mcw est. '13

	Date:	am or pm	Intervals:
	W.O.D.:	rps/rnds/lps	HrMx%
1			
2			
3			
4			
5			
6			
7			
8			
9			
10			
11			
12			
		A.L.O.I @:	

Ana/Vo2 CARDIO INTERVALS

(Hvi's) mcw est. '13

	Date:	am or pm	Intervals:
	W.O.D.:	rps/rnds/lps	HrMx%
1			
2			
3			
4			
5			
6			
7			
8			
9			
10			
11			
12			
		A.L.O.I @:	

Ana/Vo2 CARDIO INTERVALS

(Hvi's) mcw est. '13

	Date:	am or pm	Intervals:
	W.O.D.:	rps/rnds/lps	HrMx%
1			
2			
3			
4			
5			
6			
7			
8			
9			
10			
11			
12			
		A.L.O.I @:	

Ana/Vo2 CARDIO INTERVALS

(Hvi's) mcw est. '13

	Date:	am or pm	Intervals:
	W.O.D.:	rps/rnds/lps	HrMx%
1			
2			
3			
4			
5			
6			
7			
8			
9			
10			
11			
12			
		A.L.O.I @:	

Ana/Vo2 CARDIO INTERVALS

(Hvi's) mcw est. '13

	Date:	am or pm	Intervals:
	W.O.D.:	rps/rnds/lps	HrMx%
1			
2			
3			
4			
5			
6			
7			
8			
9			
10			
11			
12			
		A.L.O.I @:	

Ana/Vo2 CARDIO INTERVALS

(Hvi's) mcw est. '13

	Date:	am or pm	Intervals:
	W.O.D.:	rps/rnds/lps	HrMx%
1			
2			
3			
4			
5			
6			
7			
8			
9			
10			
11			
12			
		A.L.O.I @:	

Ana/Vo2 CARDIO INTERVALS
(Hvi's) mcw est. '13

	Date:	am or pm	Intervals:
	W.O.D.:	rps/rnds/lps	HrMx%
1			
2			
3			
4			
5			
6			
7			
8			
9			
10			
11			
12			
		A.L.O.I @:	

Ana/Vo2 CARDIO INTERVALS
(Hvi's) mcw est. '13

	Date:	am or pm	Intervals:
	W.O.D.:	rps/rnds/lps	HrMx%
1			
2			
3			
4			
5			
6			
7			
8			
9			
10			
11			
12			
		A.L.O.I @:	

Ana/Vo2 CARDIO INTERVALS
(Hvi's) mcw est. '13

	Date:	am or pm	Intervals:
	W.O.D.:	rps/rnds/lps	HrMx%
1			
2			
3			
4			
5			
6			
7			
8			
9			
10			
11			
12			
		A.L.O.I @:	

Ana/Vo2 CARDIO INTERVALS
(Hvi's) mcw est. '13

	Date:	am or pm	Intervals:
	W.O.D.:	rps/rnds/lps	HrMx%
1			
2			
3			
4			
5			
6			
7			
8			
9			
10			
11			
12			
		A.L.O.I @:	

Ana/Vo2 CARDIO INTERVALS
(Hvi's) mcw est. '13

	Date:	am or pm	Intervals:
	W.O.D.:	rps/rnds/lps	HrMx%
1			
2			
3			
4			
5			
6			
7			
8			
9			
10			
11			
12			
		A.L.O.I @:	

Ana/Vo2 CARDIO INTERVALS
(Hvi's) mcw est. '13

	Date:	am or pm	Intervals:
	W.O.D.:	rps/rnds/lps	HrMx%
1			
2			
3			
4			
5			
6			
7			
8			
9			
10			
11			
12			
		A.L.O.I @:	

FITNESS EVOLUTION NOTES:

Track your Training Effort Intensity Level Zones, Calorie Expense, and Personal Benchmark Record Data

DATE:__________ DATA:	DATE:__________ DATA:
DATE:__________ DATA:	DATE:__________ DATA:
DATE:__________ DATA:	DATE:__________ DATA:
DATE:__________ DATA:	DATE:__________ DATA:
DATE:__________ DATA:	DATE:__________ DATA:
DATE:__________ DATA:	DATE:__________ DATA:
DATE:__________ DATA:	DATE:__________ DATA:

FITNESS EVOLUTION NOTES:

Track your Training Effort Intensity Level Zones, Calorie Expense, and Personal Benchmark Record Data

DATE:__________ DATA:	DATE:__________ DATA:
DATE:__________ DATA:	DATE:__________ DATA:
DATE:__________ DATA:	DATE:__________ DATA:
DATE:__________ DATA:	DATE:__________ DATA:
DATE:__________ DATA:	DATE:__________ DATA:
DATE:__________ DATA:	DATE:__________ DATA:
DATE:__________ DATA:	DATE:__________ DATA:

NOTES:

NOTES:

6 Week Training Calendar
Month Year

SUNDAY	MONDAY	TUESDAY	WEDNESDAY	THURSDAY	FRIDAY	SATURDAY

Week 1

Date:	Date:	Date:	Date:	Date:	Date:	Date:
Mileage:	Mileage:	Mileage:	Mileage:	Mileage:	Mileage:	Mileage:

Week 2

Date:	Date:	Date:	Date:	Date:	Date:	Date:
Mileage:	Mileage:	Mileage:	Mileage:	Mileage:	Mileage:	Mileage:

Week 3

Date:	Date:	Date:	Date:	Date:	Date:	Date:
Mileage:	Mileage:	Mileage:	Mileage:	Mileage:	Mileage:	Mileage:

Week 4

Date:	Date:	Date:	Date:	Date:	Date:	Date:
Mileage:	Mileage:	Mileage:	Mileage:	Mileage:	Mileage:	Mileage:

Week 5

Date:	Date:	Date:	Date:	Date:	Date:	Date:
Mileage:	Mileage:	Mileage:	Mileage:	Mileage:	Mileage:	Mileage:

Week 6

Date:	Date:	Date:	Date:	Date:	Date:	Date:
Mileage:	Mileage:	Mileage:	Mileage:	Mileage:	Mileage:	Mileage:

Ana/Vo2 CARDIO INTERVALS
(Hvi's) mcw est. '13

	Date:	am or pm	Intervals:
	W.O.D.:	rps/rnds/lps	HrMx%
1			
2			
3			
4			
5			
6			
7			
8			
9			
10			
11			
12			
		A.L.O.I @:	

Ana/Vo2 CARDIO INTERVALS
(Hvi's) mcw est. '13

	Date:	am or pm	Intervals:
	W.O.D.:	rps/rnds/lps	HrMx%
1			
2			
3			
4			
5			
6			
7			
8			
9			
10			
11			
12			
		A.L.O.I @:	

Ana/Vo2 CARDIO INTERVALS
(Hvi's) mcw est. '13

	Date:	am or pm	Intervals:
	W.O.D.:	rps/rnds/lps	HrMx%
1			
2			
3			
4			
5			
6			
7			
8			
9			
10			
11			
12			
		A.L.O.I @:	

Ana/Vo2 CARDIO INTERVALS
(Hvi's) mcw est. '13

	Date:	am or pm	Intervals:
	W.O.D.:	rps/rnds/lps	HrMx%
1			
2			
3			
4			
5			
6			
7			
8			
9			
10			
11			
12			
		A.L.O.I @:	

Ana/Vo2 CARDIO INTERVALS
(Hvi's) mcw est. '13

	Date:	am or pm	Intervals:
	W.O.D.:	rps/rnds/lps	HrMx%
1			
2			
3			
4			
5			
6			
7			
8			
9			
10			
11			
12			
		A.L.O.I @:	

Ana/Vo2 CARDIO INTERVALS
(Hvi's) mcw est. '13

	Date:	am or pm	Intervals:
	W.O.D.:	rps/rnds/lps	HrMx%
1			
2			
3			
4			
5			
6			
7			
8			
9			
10			
11			
12			
		A.L.O.I @:	

Ana/Vo2 CARDIO INTERVALS
(Hvi's) mcw est. '13

	Date:	am or pm	Intervals:
	W.O.D.:	rps/rnds/lps	HrMx%
1			
2			
3			
4			
5			
6			
7			
8			
9			
10			
11			
12			
		A.L.O.I @:	

Ana/Vo2 CARDIO INTERVALS
(Hvi's) mcw est. '13

	Date:	am or pm	Intervals:
	W.O.D.:	rps/rnds/lps	HrMx%
1			
2			
3			
4			
5			
6			
7			
8			
9			
10			
11			
12			
		A.L.O.I @:	

Ana/Vo2 CARDIO INTERVALS
(Hvi's) mcw est. '13

	Date:	am or pm	Intervals:
	W.O.D.:	rps/rnds/lps	HrMx%
1			
2			
3			
4			
5			
6			
7			
8			
9			
10			
11			
12			
		A.L.O.I @:	

Ana/Vo2 CARDIO INTERVALS
(Hvi's) mcw est. '13

	Date:	am or pm	Intervals:
	W.O.D.:	rps/rnds/lps	HrMx%
1			
2			
3			
4			
5			
6			
7			
8			
9			
10			
11			
12			
		A.L.O.I @:	

Ana/Vo2 CARDIO INTERVALS
(Hvi's) mcw est. '13

	Date:	am or pm	Intervals:
	W.O.D.:	rps/rnds/lps	HrMx%
1			
2			
3			
4			
5			
6			
7			
8			
9			
10			
11			
12			
		A.L.O.I @:	

Ana/Vo2 CARDIO INTERVALS
(Hvi's) mcw est. '13

	Date:	am or pm	Intervals:
	W.O.D.:	rps/rnds/lps	HrMx%
1			
2			
3			
4			
5			
6			
7			
8			
9			
10			
11			
12			
		A.L.O.I @:	

Ana/Vo2 CARDIO INTERVALS

(Hvi's) mcw est. '13

	Date:	am or pm	Intervals:
	W.O.D.:	rps/rnds/lps	HrMx%
1			
2			
3			
4			
5			
6			
7			
8			
9			
10			
11			
12			
		A.L.O.I @:	

Ana/Vo2 CARDIO INTERVALS

(Hvi's) mcw est. '13

	Date:	am or pm	Intervals:
	W.O.D.:	rps/rnds/lps	HrMx%
1			
2			
3			
4			
5			
6			
7			
8			
9			
10			
11			
12			
		A.L.O.I @:	

Ana/Vo2 CARDIO INTERVALS

(Hvi's) mcw est. '13

	Date:	am or pm	Intervals:
	W.O.D.:	rps/rnds/lps	HrMx%
1			
2			
3			
4			
5			
6			
7			
8			
9			
10			
11			
12			
		A.L.O.I @:	

Ana/Vo2 CARDIO INTERVALS

(Hvi's) mcw est. '13

	Date:	am or pm	Intervals:
	W.O.D.:	rps/rnds/lps	HrMx%
1			
2			
3			
4			
5			
6			
7			
8			
9			
10			
11			
12			
		A.L.O.I @:	

Ana/Vo2 CARDIO INTERVALS

(Hvi's) mcw est. '13

	Date:	am or pm	Intervals:
	W.O.D.:	rps/rnds/lps	HrMx%
1			
2			
3			
4			
5			
6			
7			
8			
9			
10			
11			
12			
		A.L.O.I @:	

Ana/Vo2 CARDIO INTERVALS

(Hvi's) mcw est. '13

	Date:	am or pm	Intervals:
	W.O.D.:	rps/rnds/lps	HrMx%
1			
2			
3			
4			
5			
6			
7			
8			
9			
10			
11			
12			
		A.L.O.I @:	

Ana/Vo2 CARDIO INTERVALS

(Hvi's) mcw est. '13

	Date:	am or pm	Intervals:
	W.O.D.:	rps/rnds/lps	HrMx%
1			
2			
3			
4			
5			
6			
7			
8			
9			
10			
11			
12			
		A.L.O.I @:	

Ana/Vo2 CARDIO INTERVALS

(Hvi's) mcw est. '13

	Date:	am or pm	Intervals:
	W.O.D.:	rps/rnds/lps	HrMx%
1			
2			
3			
4			
5			
6			
7			
8			
9			
10			
11			
12			
		A.L.O.I @:	

Ana/Vo2 CARDIO INTERVALS

(Hvi's) mcw est. '13

	Date:	am or pm	Intervals:
	W.O.D.:	rps/rnds/lps	HrMx%
1			
2			
3			
4			
5			
6			
7			
8			
9			
10			
11			
12			
		A.L.O.I @:	

Ana/Vo2 CARDIO INTERVALS

(Hvi's) mcw est. '13

	Date:	am or pm	Intervals:
	W.O.D.:	rps/rnds/lps	HrMx%
1			
2			
3			
4			
5			
6			
7			
8			
9			
10			
11			
12			
		A.L.O.I @:	

Ana/Vo2 CARDIO INTERVALS

(Hvi's) mcw est. '13

	Date:	am or pm	Intervals:
	W.O.D.:	rps/rnds/lps	HrMx%
1			
2			
3			
4			
5			
6			
7			
8			
9			
10			
11			
12			
		A.L.O.I @:	

Ana/Vo2 CARDIO INTERVALS

(Hvi's) mcw est. '13

	Date:	am or pm	Intervals:
	W.O.D.:	rps/rnds/lps	HrMx%
1			
2			
3			
4			
5			
6			
7			
8			
9			
10			
11			
12			
		A.L.O.I @:	

Ana/Vo2 CARDIO INTERVALS

(Hvi's) mcw est. '13

	Date:	am or pm	Intervals:
	W.O.D.:	rps/rnds/lps	HrMx%
1			
2			
3			
4			
5			
6			
7			
8			
9			
10			
11			
12			
		A.L.O.I @:	

Ana/Vo2 CARDIO INTERVALS

(Hvi's) mcw est. '13

	Date:	am or pm	Intervals:
	W.O.D.:	rps/rnds/lps	HrMx%
1			
2			
3			
4			
5			
6			
7			
8			
9			
10			
11			
12			
		A.L.O.I @:	

Ana/Vo2 CARDIO INTERVALS

(Hvi's) mcw est. '13

	Date:	am or pm	Intervals:
	W.O.D.:	rps/rnds/lps	HrMx%
1			
2			
3			
4			
5			
6			
7			
8			
9			
10			
11			
12			
		A.L.O.I @:	

Ana/Vo2 CARDIO INTERVALS

(Hvi's) mcw est. '13

	Date:	am or pm	Intervals:
	W.O.D.:	rps/rnds/lps	HrMx%
1			
2			
3			
4			
5			
6			
7			
8			
9			
10			
11			
12			
		A.L.O.I @:	

Ana/Vo2 CARDIO INTERVALS

(Hvi's) mcw est. '13

	Date:	am or pm	Intervals:
	W.O.D.:	rps/rnds/lps	HrMx%
1			
2			
3			
4			
5			
6			
7			
8			
9			
10			
11			
12			
		A.L.O.I @:	

Ana/Vo2 CARDIO INTERVALS

(Hvi's) mcw est. '13

	Date:	am or pm	Intervals:
	W.O.D.:	rps/rnds/lps	HrMx%
1			
2			
3			
4			
5			
6			
7			
8			
9			
10			
11			
12			
		A.L.O.I @:	

FITNESS EVOLUTION NOTES:

Track your Training Effort Intensity Level Zones, Calorie Expense, and Personal Benchmark Record Data

DATE:____________ DATA:	DATE:____________ DATA:
DATE:____________ DATA:	DATE:____________ DATA:
DATE:____________ DATA:	DATE:____________ DATA:
DATE:____________ DATA:	DATE:____________ DATA:
DATE:____________ DATA:	DATE:____________ DATA:
DATE:____________ DATA:	DATE:____________ DATA:
DATE:____________ DATA:	DATE:____________ DATA:

FITNESS EVOLUTION NOTES:

Track your Training Effort Intensity Level Zones, Calorie Expense, and Personal Benchmark Record Data

DATE:________ DATA:	DATE:________ DATA:
DATE:________ DATA:	DATE:________ DATA:
DATE:________ DATA:	DATE:________ DATA:
DATE:________ DATA:	DATE:________ DATA:
DATE:________ DATA:	DATE:________ DATA:
DATE:________ DATA:	DATE:________ DATA:
DATE:________ DATA:	DATE:________ DATA:

NOTES:

NOTES:

6 Week Training Calendar

Month Year

SUNDAY	MONDAY	TUESDAY	WEDNESDAY	THURSDAY	FRIDAY	SATURDAY

Week 1

Date:	Date:	Date:	Date:	Date:	Date:	Date:
Mileage:	Mileage:	Mileage:	Mileage:	Mileage:	Mileage:	Mileage:

Week 2

Date:	Date:	Date:	Date:	Date:	Date:	Date:
Mileage:	Mileage:	Mileage:	Mileage:	Mileage:	Mileage:	Mileage:

Week 3

Date:	Date:	Date:	Date:	Date:	Date:	Date:
Mileage:	Mileage:	Mileage:	Mileage:	Mileage:	Mileage:	Mileage:

Week 4

Date:	Date:	Date:	Date:	Date:	Date:	Date:
Mileage:	Mileage:	Mileage:	Mileage:	Mileage:	Mileage:	Mileage:

Week 5

Date:	Date:	Date:	Date:	Date:	Date:	Date:
Mileage:	Mileage:	Mileage:	Mileage:	Mileage:	Mileage:	Mileage:

Week 6

Date:	Date:	Date:	Date:	Date:	Date:	Date:
Mileage:	Mileage:	Mileage:	Mileage:	Mileage:	Mileage:	Mileage:

Ana/Vo2 CARDIO INTERVALS

(Hvi's) mcw est. '13

	Date:	am or pm	Intervals:
	W.O.D.:	rps/rnds/lps	HrMx%
1			
2			
3			
4			
5			
6			
7			
8			
9			
10			
11			
12			
		A.L.O.I @:	

Ana/Vo2 CARDIO INTERVALS

(Hvi's) mcw est. '13

	Date:	am or pm	Intervals:
	W.O.D.:	rps/rnds/lps	HrMx%
1			
2			
3			
4			
5			
6			
7			
8			
9			
10			
11			
12			
		A.L.O.I @:	

Ana/Vo2 CARDIO INTERVALS

(Hvi's) mcw est. '13

	Date:	am or pm	Intervals:
	W.O.D.:	rps/rnds/lps	HrMx%
1			
2			
3			
4			
5			
6			
7			
8			
9			
10			
11			
12			
		A.L.O.I @:	

Ana/Vo2 CARDIO INTERVALS

(Hvi's) mcw est. '13

	Date:	am or pm	Intervals:
	W.O.D.:	rps/rnds/lps	HrMx%
1			
2			
3			
4			
5			
6			
7			
8			
9			
10			
11			
12			
		A.L.O.I @:	

Ana/Vo2 CARDIO INTERVALS

(Hvi's) mcw est. '13

	Date:	am or pm	Intervals:
	W.O.D.:	rps/rnds/lps	HrMx%
1			
2			
3			
4			
5			
6			
7			
8			
9			
10			
11			
12			
		A.L.O.I @:	

Ana/Vo2 CARDIO INTERVALS

(Hvi's) mcw est. '13

	Date:	am or pm	Intervals:
	W.O.D.:	rps/rnds/lps	HrMx%
1			
2			
3			
4			
5			
6			
7			
8			
9			
10			
11			
12			
		A.L.O.I @:	

Ana/Vo2 CARDIO INTERVALS

(Hvi's) mcw est. '13

	Date:	am or pm	Intervals:
	W.O.D.:	rps/rnds/lps	HrMx%
1			
2			
3			
4			
5			
6			
7			
8			
9			
10			
11			
12			
		A.L.O.I @:	

Ana/Vo2 CARDIO INTERVALS

(Hvi's) mcw est. '13

	Date:	am or pm	Intervals:
	W.O.D.:	rps/rnds/lps	HrMx%
1			
2			
3			
4			
5			
6			
7			
8			
9			
10			
11			
12			
		A.L.O.I @:	

Ana/Vo2 CARDIO INTERVALS

(Hvi's) mcw est. '13

	Date:	am or pm	Intervals:
	W.O.D.:	rps/rnds/lps	HrMx%
1			
2			
3			
4			
5			
6			
7			
8			
9			
10			
11			
12			
		A.L.O.I @:	

Ana/Vo2 CARDIO INTERVALS

(Hvi's) mcw est. '13

	Date:	am or pm	Intervals:
	W.O.D.:	rps/rnds/lps	HrMx%
1			
2			
3			
4			
5			
6			
7			
8			
9			
10			
11			
12			
		A.L.O.I @:	

Ana/Vo2 CARDIO INTERVALS

(Hvi's) mcw est. '13

	Date:	am or pm	Intervals:
	W.O.D.:	rps/rnds/lps	HrMx%
1			
2			
3			
4			
5			
6			
7			
8			
9			
10			
11			
12			
		A.L.O.I @:	

Ana/Vo2 CARDIO INTERVALS

(Hvi's) mcw est. '13

	Date:	am or pm	Intervals:
	W.O.D.:	rps/rnds/lps	HrMx%
1			
2			
3			
4			
5			
6			
7			
8			
9			
10			
11			
12			
		A.L.O.I @:	

Ana/Vo2 CARDIO INTERVALS

(Hvi's) mcw est. '13

	Date:	am or pm	Intervals:
	W.O.D.:	rps/rnds/lps	HrMx%
1			
2			
3			
4			
5			
6			
7			
8			
9			
10			
11			
12			
		A.L.O.I @:	

Ana/Vo2 CARDIO INTERVALS

(Hvi's) mcw est. '13

	Date:	am or pm	Intervals:
	W.O.D.:	rps/rnds/lps	HrMx%
1			
2			
3			
4			
5			
6			
7			
8			
9			
10			
11			
12			
		A.L.O.I @:	

Ana/Vo2 CARDIO INTERVALS

(Hvi's) mcw est. '13

	Date:	am or pm	Intervals:
	W.O.D.:	rps/rnds/lps	HrMx%
1			
2			
3			
4			
5			
6			
7			
8			
9			
10			
11			
12			
		A.L.O.I @:	

Ana/Vo2 CARDIO INTERVALS

(Hvi's) mcw est. '13

	Date:	am or pm	Intervals:
	W.O.D.:	rps/rnds/lps	HrMx%
1			
2			
3			
4			
5			
6			
7			
8			
9			
10			
11			
12			
		A.L.O.I @:	

Ana/Vo2 CARDIO INTERVALS

(Hvi's) mcw est. '13

	Date:	am or pm	Intervals:
	W.O.D.:	rps/rnds/lps	HrMx%
1			
2			
3			
4			
5			
6			
7			
8			
9			
10			
11			
12			
		A.L.O.I @:	

Ana/Vo2 CARDIO INTERVALS

(Hvi's) mcw est. '13

	Date:	am or pm	Intervals:
	W.O.D.:	rps/rnds/lps	HrMx%
1			
2			
3			
4			
5			
6			
7			
8			
9			
10			
11			
12			
		A.L.O.I @:	

Ana/Vo2 CARDIO INTERVALS

(Hvi's) mcw est. '13

	Date:	am or pm	Intervals:
	W.O.D.:	rps/rnds/lps	HrMx%
1			
2			
3			
4			
5			
6			
7			
8			
9			
10			
11			
12			
		A.L.O.I @:	

Ana/Vo2 CARDIO INTERVALS

(Hvi's) mcw est. '13

	Date:	am or pm	Intervals:
	W.O.D.:	rps/rnds/lps	HrMx%
1			
2			
3			
4			
5			
6			
7			
8			
9			
10			
11			
12			
		A.L.O.I @:	

Ana/Vo2 CARDIO INTERVALS

(Hvi's) mcw est. '13

	Date:	am or pm	Intervals:
	W.O.D.:	rps/rnds/lps	HrMx%
1			
2			
3			
4			
5			
6			
7			
8			
9			
10			
11			
12			
		A.L.O.I @:	

Ana/Vo2 CARDIO INTERVALS

(Hvi's) mcw est. '13

	Date:	am or pm	Intervals:
	W.O.D.:	rps/rnds/lps	HrMx%
1			
2			
3			
4			
5			
6			
7			
8			
9			
10			
11			
12			
		A.L.O.I @:	

Ana/Vo2 CARDIO INTERVALS

(Hvi's) mcw est. '13

	Date:	am or pm	Intervals:
	W.O.D.:	rps/rnds/lps	HrMx%
1			
2			
3			
4			
5			
6			
7			
8			
9			
10			
11			
12			
		A.L.O.I @:	

Ana/Vo2 CARDIO INTERVALS

(Hvi's) mcw est. '13

	Date:	am or pm	Intervals:
	W.O.D.:	rps/rnds/lps	HrMx%
1			
2			
3			
4			
5			
6			
7			
8			
9			
10			
11			
12			
		A.L.O.I @:	

Ana/Vo2 CARDIO INTERVALS

(Hvi's) mcw est. '13

	Date:	am or pm	Intervals:
	W.O.D.:	rps/rnds/lps	HrMx%
1			
2			
3			
4			
5			
6			
7			
8			
9			
10			
11			
12			
		A.L.O.I @:	

Ana/Vo2 CARDIO INTERVALS

(Hvi's) mcw est. '13

	Date:	am or pm	Intervals:
	W.O.D.:	rps/rnds/lps	HrMx%
1			
2			
3			
4			
5			
6			
7			
8			
9			
10			
11			
12			
		A.L.O.I @:	

Ana/Vo2 CARDIO INTERVALS

(Hvi's) mcw est. '13

	Date:	am or pm	Intervals:
	W.O.D.:	rps/rnds/lps	HrMx%
1			
2			
3			
4			
5			
6			
7			
8			
9			
10			
11			
12			
		A.L.O.I @:	

Ana/Vo2 CARDIO INTERVALS

(Hvi's) mcw est. '13

	Date:	am or pm	Intervals:
	W.O.D.:	rps/rnds/lps	HrMx%
1			
2			
3			
4			
5			
6			
7			
8			
9			
10			
11			
12			
		A.L.O.I @:	

Ana/Vo2 CARDIO INTERVALS

(Hvi's) mcw est. '13

	Date:	am or pm	Intervals:
	W.O.D.:	rps/rnds/lps	HrMx%
1			
2			
3			
4			
5			
6			
7			
8			
9			
10			
11			
12			
		A.L.O.I @:	

Ana/Vo2 CARDIO INTERVALS

(Hvi's) mcw est. '13

	Date:	am or pm	Intervals:
	W.O.D.:	rps/rnds/lps	HrMx%
1			
2			
3			
4			
5			
6			
7			
8			
9			
10			
11			
12			
		A.L.O.I @:	

FITNESS EVOLUTION NOTES:

Track your Training Effort Intensity Level Zones, Calorie Expense, and Personal Benchmark Record Data

DATE:__________ DATA:	DATE:__________ DATA:
DATE:__________ DATA:	DATE:__________ DATA:
DATE:__________ DATA:	DATE:__________ DATA:
DATE:__________ DATA:	DATE:__________ DATA:
DATE:__________ DATA:	DATE:__________ DATA:
DATE:__________ DATA:	DATE:__________ DATA:
DATE:__________ DATA:	DATE:__________ DATA:

FITNESS EVOLUTION NOTES:

Track your Training Effort Intensity Level Zones, Calorie Expense, and Personal Benchmark Record Data

DATE:__________ DATA:	DATE:__________ DATA:
DATE:__________ DATA:	DATE:__________ DATA:
DATE:__________ DATA:	DATE:__________ DATA:
DATE:__________ DATA:	DATE:__________ DATA:
DATE:__________ DATA:	DATE:__________ DATA:
DATE:__________ DATA:	DATE:__________ DATA:
DATE:__________ DATA:	DATE:__________ DATA:

NOTES:

NOTES:

6 Week Training Calendar

Month Year

SUNDAY	MONDAY	TUESDAY	WEDNESDAY	THURSDAY	FRIDAY	SATURDAY

Week 1

Date:	Date:	Date:	Date:	Date:	Date:	Date:
Mileage:	Mileage:	Mileage:	Mileage:	Mileage:	Mileage:	Mileage:

Week 2

Date:	Date:	Date:	Date:	Date:	Date:	Date:
Mileage:	Mileage:	Mileage:	Mileage:	Mileage:	Mileage:	Mileage:

Week 3

Date:	Date:	Date:	Date:	Date:	Date:	Date:
Mileage:	Mileage:	Mileage:	Mileage:	Mileage:	Mileage:	Mileage:

Week 4

Date:	Date:	Date:	Date:	Date:	Date:	Date:
Mileage:	Mileage:	Mileage:	Mileage:	Mileage:	Mileage:	Mileage:

Week 5

Date:	Date:	Date:	Date:	Date:	Date:	Date:
Mileage:	Mileage:	Mileage:	Mileage:	Mileage:	Mileage:	Mileage:

Week 6

Date:	Date:	Date:	Date:	Date:	Date:	Date:
Mileage:	Mileage:	Mileage:	Mileage:	Mileage:	Mileage:	Mileage:

Ana/Vo2 CARDIO INTERVALS

(Hvi's) mcw est. '13

	Date:	am or pm	Intervals:
	W.O.D.:	rps/rnds/lps	HrMx%
1			
2			
3			
4			
5			
6			
7			
8			
9			
10			
11			
12			
		A.L.O.I @:	

Ana/Vo2 CARDIO INTERVALS

(Hvi's) mcw est. '13

	Date:	am or pm	Intervals:
	W.O.D.:	rps/rnds/lps	HrMx%
1			
2			
3			
4			
5			
6			
7			
8			
9			
10			
11			
12			
		A.L.O.I @:	

Ana/Vo2 CARDIO INTERVALS

(Hvi's) mcw est. '13

	Date:	am or pm	Intervals:
	W.O.D.:	rps/rnds/lps	HrMx%
1			
2			
3			
4			
5			
6			
7			
8			
9			
10			
11			
12			
		A.L.O.I @:	

Ana/Vo2 CARDIO INTERVALS

(Hvi's) mcw est. '13

	Date:	am or pm	Intervals:
	W.O.D.:	rps/rnds/lps	HrMx%
1			
2			
3			
4			
5			
6			
7			
8			
9			
10			
11			
12			
		A.L.O.I @:	

Ana/Vo2 CARDIO INTERVALS

(Hvi's) mcw est. '13

	Date:	am or pm	Intervals:
	W.O.D.:	rps/rnds/lps	HrMx%
1			
2			
3			
4			
5			
6			
7			
8			
9			
10			
11			
12			
		A.L.O.I @:	

Ana/Vo2 CARDIO INTERVALS

(Hvi's) mcw est. '13

	Date:	am or pm	Intervals:
	W.O.D.:	rps/rnds/lps	HrMx%
1			
2			
3			
4			
5			
6			
7			
8			
9			
10			
11			
12			
		A.L.O.I @:	

Ana/Vo2 CARDIO INTERVALS

(Hvi's) mcw est. '13

Date:	am or pm	Intervals:
W.O.D.:	rps/rnds/lps	HrMx%
1		
2		
3		
4		
5		
6		
7		
8		
9		
10		
11		
12		
	A.L.O.I @:	

Ana/Vo2 CARDIO INTERVALS

(Hvi's) mcw est. '13

Date:	am or pm	Intervals:
W.O.D.:	rps/rnds/lps	HrMx%
1		
2		
3		
4		
5		
6		
7		
8		
9		
10		
11		
12		
	A.L.O.I @:	

Ana/Vo2 CARDIO INTERVALS

(Hvi's) mcw est. '13

Date:	am or pm	Intervals:
W.O.D.:	rps/rnds/lps	HrMx%
1		
2		
3		
4		
5		
6		
7		
8		
9		
10		
11		
12		
	A.L.O.I @:	

Ana/Vo2 CARDIO INTERVALS

(Hvi's) mcw est. '13

Date:	am or pm	Intervals:
W.O.D.:	rps/rnds/lps	HrMx%
1		
2		
3		
4		
5		
6		
7		
8		
9		
10		
11		
12		
	A.L.O.I @:	

Ana/Vo2 CARDIO INTERVALS

(Hvi's) mcw est. '13

Date:	am or pm	Intervals:
W.O.D.:	rps/rnds/lps	HrMx%
1		
2		
3		
4		
5		
6		
7		
8		
9		
10		
11		
12		
	A.L.O.I @:	

Ana/Vo2 CARDIO INTERVALS

(Hvi's) mcw est. '13

Date:	am or pm	Intervals:
W.O.D.:	rps/rnds/lps	HrMx%
1		
2		
3		
4		
5		
6		
7		
8		
9		
10		
11		
12		
	A.L.O.I @:	

Ana/Vo2 CARDIO INTERVALS
(Hvi's) mcw est. '13

	Date:	am or pm	Intervals:
	W.O.D.:	rps/rnds/lps	HrMx%
1			
2			
3			
4			
5			
6			
7			
8			
9			
10			
11			
12			
		A.L.O.I @:	

Ana/Vo2 CARDIO INTERVALS
(Hvi's) mcw est. '13

	Date:	am or pm	Intervals:
	W.O.D.:	rps/rnds/lps	HrMx%
1			
2			
3			
4			
5			
6			
7			
8			
9			
10			
11			
12			
		A.L.O.I @:	

Ana/Vo2 CARDIO INTERVALS
(Hvi's) mcw est. '13

	Date:	am or pm	Intervals:
	W.O.D.:	rps/rnds/lps	HrMx%
1			
2			
3			
4			
5			
6			
7			
8			
9			
10			
11			
12			
		A.L.O.I @:	

Ana/Vo2 CARDIO INTERVALS
(Hvi's) mcw est. '13

	Date:	am or pm	Intervals:
	W.O.D.:	rps/rnds/lps	HrMx%
1			
2			
3			
4			
5			
6			
7			
8			
9			
10			
11			
12			
		A.L.O.I @:	

Ana/Vo2 CARDIO INTERVALS
(Hvi's) mcw est. '13

	Date:	am or pm	Intervals:
	W.O.D.:	rps/rnds/lps	HrMx%
1			
2			
3			
4			
5			
6			
7			
8			
9			
10			
11			
12			
		A.L.O.I @:	

Ana/Vo2 CARDIO INTERVALS
(Hvi's) mcw est. '13

	Date:	am or pm	Intervals:
	W.O.D.:	rps/rnds/lps	HrMx%
1			
2			
3			
4			
5			
6			
7			
8			
9			
10			
11			
12			
		A.L.O.I @:	

Ana/Vo2 CARDIO INTERVALS
(Hvi's) mcw est. '13

Date:	am or pm	Intervals:
W.O.D.:	rps/rnds/lps	HrMx%
1		
2		
3		
4		
5		
6		
7		
8		
9		
10		
11		
12		
	A.L.O.I @:	

Ana/Vo2 CARDIO INTERVALS
(Hvi's) mcw est. '13

Date:	am or pm	Intervals:
W.O.D.:	rps/rnds/lps	HrMx%
1		
2		
3		
4		
5		
6		
7		
8		
9		
10		
11		
12		
	A.L.O.I @:	

Ana/Vo2 CARDIO INTERVALS
(Hvi's) mcw est. '13

Date:	am or pm	Intervals:
W.O.D.:	rps/rnds/lps	HrMx%
1		
2		
3		
4		
5		
6		
7		
8		
9		
10		
11		
12		
	A.L.O.I @:	

Ana/Vo2 CARDIO INTERVALS
(Hvi's) mcw est. '13

Date:	am or pm	Intervals:
W.O.D.:	rps/rnds/lps	HrMx%
1		
2		
3		
4		
5		
6		
7		
8		
9		
10		
11		
12		
	A.L.O.I @:	

Ana/Vo2 CARDIO INTERVALS
(Hvi's) mcw est. '13

Date:	am or pm	Intervals:
W.O.D.:	rps/rnds/lps	HrMx%
1		
2		
3		
4		
5		
6		
7		
8		
9		
10		
11		
12		
	A.L.O.I @:	

Ana/Vo2 CARDIO INTERVALS
(Hvi's) mcw est. '13

Date:	am or pm	Intervals:
W.O.D.:	rps/rnds/lps	HrMx%
1		
2		
3		
4		
5		
6		
7		
8		
9		
10		
11		
12		
	A.L.O.I @:	

Ana/Vo2 CARDIO INTERVALS
(Hvi's) mcw est. '13

	Date:	am or pm	Intervals:
	W.O.D.:	rps/rnds/lps	HrMx%
1			
2			
3			
4			
5			
6			
7			
8			
9			
10			
11			
12			
		A.L.O.I @:	

Ana/Vo2 CARDIO INTERVALS
(Hvi's) mcw est. '13

	Date:	am or pm	Intervals:
	W.O.D.:	rps/rnds/lps	HrMx%
1			
2			
3			
4			
5			
6			
7			
8			
9			
10			
11			
12			
		A.L.O.I @:	

Ana/Vo2 CARDIO INTERVALS
(Hvi's) mcw est. '13

	Date:	am or pm	Intervals:
	W.O.D.:	rps/rnds/lps	HrMx%
1			
2			
3			
4			
5			
6			
7			
8			
9			
10			
11			
12			
		A.L.O.I @:	

Ana/Vo2 CARDIO INTERVALS
(Hvi's) mcw est. '13

	Date:	am or pm	Intervals:
	W.O.D.:	rps/rnds/lps	HrMx%
1			
2			
3			
4			
5			
6			
7			
8			
9			
10			
11			
12			
		A.L.O.I @:	

Ana/Vo2 CARDIO INTERVALS
(Hvi's) mcw est. '13

	Date:	am or pm	Intervals:
	W.O.D.:	rps/rnds/lps	HrMx%
1			
2			
3			
4			
5			
6			
7			
8			
9			
10			
11			
12			
		A.L.O.I @:	

Ana/Vo2 CARDIO INTERVALS
(Hvi's) mcw est. '13

	Date:	am or pm	Intervals:
	W.O.D.:	rps/rnds/lps	HrMx%
1			
2			
3			
4			
5			
6			
7			
8			
9			
10			
11			
12			
		A.L.O.I @:	

FITNESS EVOLUTION NOTES:

Track your Training Effort Intensity Level Zones, Calorie Expense, and Personal Benchmark Record Data

DATE:__________ DATA:	DATE:__________ DATA:
DATE:__________ DATA:	DATE:__________ DATA:
DATE:__________ DATA:	DATE:__________ DATA:
DATE:__________ DATA:	DATE:__________ DATA:
DATE:__________ DATA:	DATE:__________ DATA:
DATE:__________ DATA:	DATE:__________ DATA:
DATE:__________ DATA:	DATE:__________ DATA:

FITNESS EVOLUTION NOTES:

Track your Training Effort Intensity Level Zones, Calorie Expense, and Personal Benchmark Record Data

DATE:________ DATA:	DATE:________ DATA:
DATE:________ DATA:	DATE:________ DATA:
DATE:________ DATA:	DATE:________ DATA:
DATE:________ DATA:	DATE:________ DATA:
DATE:________ DATA:	DATE:________ DATA:
DATE:________ DATA:	DATE:________ DATA:
DATE:________ DATA:	DATE:________ DATA:

NOTES:

NOTES:

6 Week Training Calendar

Month Year

SUNDAY	MONDAY	TUESDAY	WEDNESDAY	THURSDAY	FRIDAY	SATURDAY

Week 1

Date:	Date:	Date:	Date:	Date:	Date:	Date:
Mileage:	Mileage:	Mileage:	Mileage:	Mileage:	Mileage:	Mileage:

Week 2

Date:	Date:	Date:	Date:	Date:	Date:	Date:
Mileage:	Mileage:	Mileage:	Mileage:	Mileage:	Mileage:	Mileage:

Week 3

Date:	Date:	Date:	Date:	Date:	Date:	Date:
Mileage:	Mileage:	Mileage:	Mileage:	Mileage:	Mileage:	Mileage:

Week 4

Date:	Date:	Date:	Date:	Date:	Date:	Date:
Mileage:	Mileage:	Mileage:	Mileage:	Mileage:	Mileage:	Mileage:

Week 5

Date:	Date:	Date:	Date:	Date:	Date:	Date:
Mileage:	Mileage:	Mileage:	Mileage:	Mileage:	Mileage:	Mileage:

Week 6

Date:	Date:	Date:	Date:	Date:	Date:	Date:
Mileage:	Mileage:	Mileage:	Mileage:	Mileage:	Mileage:	Mileage:

Ana/Vo2 CARDIO INTERVALS

(Hvi's) mcw est. '13

	Date:	am or pm	Intervals:
	W.O.D.:	rps/rnds/lps	HrMx%
1			
2			
3			
4			
5			
6			
7			
8			
9			
10			
11			
12			
		A.L.O.I @:	

Ana/Vo2 CARDIO INTERVALS

(Hvi's) mcw est. '13

	Date:	am or pm	Intervals:
	W.O.D.:	rps/rnds/lps	HrMx%
1			
2			
3			
4			
5			
6			
7			
8			
9			
10			
11			
12			
		A.L.O.I @:	

Ana/Vo2 CARDIO INTERVALS

(Hvi's) mcw est. '13

	Date:	am or pm	Intervals:
	W.O.D.:	rps/rnds/lps	HrMx%
1			
2			
3			
4			
5			
6			
7			
8			
9			
10			
11			
12			
		A.L.O.I @:	

Ana/Vo2 CARDIO INTERVALS

(Hvi's) mcw est. '13

	Date:	am or pm	Intervals:
	W.O.D.:	rps/rnds/lps	HrMx%
1			
2			
3			
4			
5			
6			
7			
8			
9			
10			
11			
12			
		A.L.O.I @:	

Ana/Vo2 CARDIO INTERVALS

(Hvi's) mcw est. '13

	Date:	am or pm	Intervals:
	W.O.D.:	rps/rnds/lps	HrMx%
1			
2			
3			
4			
5			
6			
7			
8			
9			
10			
11			
12			
		A.L.O.I @:	

Ana/Vo2 CARDIO INTERVALS

(Hvi's) mcw est. '13

	Date:	am or pm	Intervals:
	W.O.D.:	rps/rnds/lps	HrMx%
1			
2			
3			
4			
5			
6			
7			
8			
9			
10			
11			
12			
		A.L.O.I @:	

Ana/Vo2 CARDIO INTERVALS

(Hvi's) mcw est. '13

	Date:	am or pm	Intervals:
	W.O.D.:	rps/rnds/lps	HrMx%
1			
2			
3			
4			
5			
6			
7			
8			
9			
10			
11			
12			

A.L.O.I @:

Ana/Vo2 CARDIO INTERVALS

(Hvi's) mcw est. '13

	Date:	am or pm	Intervals:
	W.O.D.:	rps/rnds/lps	HrMx%
1			
2			
3			
4			
5			
6			
7			
8			
9			
10			
11			
12			

A.L.O.I @:

Ana/Vo2 CARDIO INTERVALS

(Hvi's) mcw est. '13

	Date:	am or pm	Intervals:
	W.O.D.:	rps/rnds/lps	HrMx%
1			
2			
3			
4			
5			
6			
7			
8			
9			
10			
11			
12			

A.L.O.I @:

Ana/Vo2 CARDIO INTERVALS

(Hvi's) mcw est. '13

	Date:	am or pm	Intervals:
	W.O.D.:	rps/rnds/lps	HrMx%
1			
2			
3			
4			
5			
6			
7			
8			
9			
10			
11			
12			

A.L.O.I @:

Ana/Vo2 CARDIO INTERVALS

(Hvi's) mcw est. '13

	Date:	am or pm	Intervals:
	W.O.D.:	rps/rnds/lps	HrMx%
1			
2			
3			
4			
5			
6			
7			
8			
9			
10			
11			
12			

A.L.O.I @:

Ana/Vo2 CARDIO INTERVALS

(Hvi's) mcw est. '13

	Date:	am or pm	Intervals:
	W.O.D.:	rps/rnds/lps	HrMx%
1			
2			
3			
4			
5			
6			
7			
8			
9			
10			
11			
12			

A.L.O.I @:

Ana/Vo2 CARDIO INTERVALS
(Hvi's) mcw est. '13

	Date:	am or pm	Intervals:
	W.O.D.:	rps/rnds/lps	HrMx%
1			
2			
3			
4			
5			
6			
7			
8			
9			
10			
11			
12			
		A.L.O.I @:	

Ana/Vo2 CARDIO INTERVALS
(Hvi's) mcw est. '13

	Date:	am or pm	Intervals:
	W.O.D.:	rps/rnds/lps	HrMx%
1			
2			
3			
4			
5			
6			
7			
8			
9			
10			
11			
12			
		A.L.O.I @:	

Ana/Vo2 CARDIO INTERVALS
(Hvi's) mcw est. '13

	Date:	am or pm	Intervals:
	W.O.D.:	rps/rnds/lps	HrMx%
1			
2			
3			
4			
5			
6			
7			
8			
9			
10			
11			
12			
		A.L.O.I @:	

Ana/Vo2 CARDIO INTERVALS
(Hvi's) mcw est. '13

	Date:	am or pm	Intervals:
	W.O.D.:	rps/rnds/lps	HrMx%
1			
2			
3			
4			
5			
6			
7			
8			
9			
10			
11			
12			
		A.L.O.I @:	

Ana/Vo2 CARDIO INTERVALS
(Hvi's) mcw est. '13

	Date:	am or pm	Intervals:
	W.O.D.:	rps/rnds/lps	HrMx%
1			
2			
3			
4			
5			
6			
7			
8			
9			
10			
11			
12			
		A.L.O.I @:	

Ana/Vo2 CARDIO INTERVALS
(Hvi's) mcw est. '13

	Date:	am or pm	Intervals:
	W.O.D.:	rps/rnds/lps	HrMx%
1			
2			
3			
4			
5			
6			
7			
8			
9			
10			
11			
12			
		A.L.O.I @:	

Ana/Vo2 CARDIO INTERVALS
(Hvi's) mcw est. '13

	Date:	am or pm	Intervals:
	W.O.D.:	rps/rnds/lps	HrMx%
1			
2			
3			
4			
5			
6			
7			
8			
9			
10			
11			
12			
		A.L.O.I @:	

Ana/Vo2 CARDIO INTERVALS
(Hvi's) mcw est. '13

	Date:	am or pm	Intervals:
	W.O.D.:	rps/rnds/lps	HrMx%
1			
2			
3			
4			
5			
6			
7			
8			
9			
10			
11			
12			
		A.L.O.I @:	

Ana/Vo2 CARDIO INTERVALS
(Hvi's) mcw est. '13

	Date:	am or pm	Intervals:
	W.O.D.:	rps/rnds/lps	HrMx%
1			
2			
3			
4			
5			
6			
7			
8			
9			
10			
11			
12			
		A.L.O.I @:	

Ana/Vo2 CARDIO INTERVALS
(Hvi's) mcw est. '13

	Date:	am or pm	Intervals:
	W.O.D.:	rps/rnds/lps	HrMx%
1			
2			
3			
4			
5			
6			
7			
8			
9			
10			
11			
12			
		A.L.O.I @:	

Ana/Vo2 CARDIO INTERVALS
(Hvi's) mcw est. '13

	Date:	am or pm	Intervals:
	W.O.D.:	rps/rnds/lps	HrMx%
1			
2			
3			
4			
5			
6			
7			
8			
9			
10			
11			
12			
		A.L.O.I @:	

Ana/Vo2 CARDIO INTERVALS
(Hvi's) mcw est. '13

	Date:	am or pm	Intervals:
	W.O.D.:	rps/rnds/lps	HrMx%
1			
2			
3			
4			
5			
6			
7			
8			
9			
10			
11			
12			
		A.L.O.I @:	

Ana/Vo2 CARDIO INTERVALS

(Hvi's) mcw est. '13

	Date:	am or pm	Intervals:
	W.O.D.:	rps/rnds/lps	HrMx%
1			
2			
3			
4			
5			
6			
7			
8			
9			
10			
11			
12			
		A.L.O.I @:	

Ana/Vo2 CARDIO INTERVALS

(Hvi's) mcw est. '13

	Date:	am or pm	Intervals:
	W.O.D.:	rps/rnds/lps	HrMx%
1			
2			
3			
4			
5			
6			
7			
8			
9			
10			
11			
12			
		A.L.O.I @:	

Ana/Vo2 CARDIO INTERVALS

(Hvi's) mcw est. '13

	Date:	am or pm	Intervals:
	W.O.D.:	rps/rnds/lps	HrMx%
1			
2			
3			
4			
5			
6			
7			
8			
9			
10			
11			
12			
		A.L.O.I @:	

Ana/Vo2 CARDIO INTERVALS

(Hvi's) mcw est. '13

	Date:	am or pm	Intervals:
	W.O.D.:	rps/rnds/lps	HrMx%
1			
2			
3			
4			
5			
6			
7			
8			
9			
10			
11			
12			
		A.L.O.I @:	

Ana/Vo2 CARDIO INTERVALS

(Hvi's) mcw est. '13

	Date:	am or pm	Intervals:
	W.O.D.:	rps/rnds/lps	HrMx%
1			
2			
3			
4			
5			
6			
7			
8			
9			
10			
11			
12			
		A.L.O.I @:	

Ana/Vo2 CARDIO INTERVALS

(Hvi's) mcw est. '13

	Date:	am or pm	Intervals:
	W.O.D.:	rps/rnds/lps	HrMx%
1			
2			
3			
4			
5			
6			
7			
8			
9			
10			
11			
12			
		A.L.O.I @:	

FITNESS EVOLUTION NOTES:

Track your Training Effort Intensity Level Zones, Calorie Expense, and Personal Benchmark Record Data

DATE:__________ DATA:	DATE:__________ DATA:
DATE:__________ DATA:	DATE:__________ DATA:
DATE:__________ DATA:	DATE:__________ DATA:
DATE:__________ DATA:	DATE:__________ DATA:
DATE:__________ DATA:	DATE:__________ DATA:
DATE:__________ DATA:	DATE:__________ DATA:
DATE:__________ DATA:	DATE:__________ DATA:

FITNESS EVOLUTION NOTES:

Track your Training Effort Intensity Level Zones, Calorie Expense, and Personal Benchmark Record Data

DATE:________ DATA:	DATE:________ DATA:
DATE:________ DATA:	DATE:________ DATA:
DATE:________ DATA:	DATE:________ DATA:
DATE:________ DATA:	DATE:________ DATA:
DATE:________ DATA:	DATE:________ DATA:
DATE:________ DATA:	DATE:________ DATA:
DATE:________ DATA:	DATE:________ DATA:

NOTES:

NOTES:

6 Week Training Calendar
Month Year

SUNDAY	MONDAY	TUESDAY	WEDNESDAY	THURSDAY	FRIDAY	SATURDAY

Week 1

Date:	Date:	Date:	Date:	Date:	Date:	Date:
Mileage:	Mileage:	Mileage:	Mileage:	Mileage:	Mileage:	Mileage:

Week 2

Date:	Date:	Date:	Date:	Date:	Date:	Date:
Mileage:	Mileage:	Mileage:	Mileage:	Mileage:	Mileage:	Mileage:

Week 3

Date:	Date:	Date:	Date:	Date:	Date:	Date:
Mileage:	Mileage:	Mileage:	Mileage:	Mileage:	Mileage:	Mileage:

Week 4

Date:	Date:	Date:	Date:	Date:	Date:	Date:
Mileage:	Mileage:	Mileage:	Mileage:	Mileage:	Mileage:	Mileage:

Week 5

Date:	Date:	Date:	Date:	Date:	Date:	Date:
Mileage:	Mileage:	Mileage:	Mileage:	Mileage:	Mileage:	Mileage:

Week 6

Date:	Date:	Date:	Date:	Date:	Date:	Date:
Mileage:	Mileage:	Mileage:	Mileage:	Mileage:	Mileage:	Mileage:

Ana/Vo2 CARDIO INTERVALS

(Hvi's) mcw est. '13

	Date:	am or pm	Intervals:
	W.O.D.:	rps/rnds/lps	HrMx%
1			
2			
3			
4			
5			
6			
7			
8			
9			
10			
11			
12			
		A.L.O.I @:	

Ana/Vo2 CARDIO INTERVALS

(Hvi's) mcw est. '13

	Date:	am or pm	Intervals:
	W.O.D.:	rps/rnds/lps	HrMx%
1			
2			
3			
4			
5			
6			
7			
8			
9			
10			
11			
12			
		A.L.O.I @:	

Ana/Vo2 CARDIO INTERVALS

(Hvi's) mcw est. '13

	Date:	am or pm	Intervals:
	W.O.D.:	rps/rnds/lps	HrMx%
1			
2			
3			
4			
5			
6			
7			
8			
9			
10			
11			
12			
		A.L.O.I @:	

Ana/Vo2 CARDIO INTERVALS

(Hvi's) mcw est. '13

	Date:	am or pm	Intervals:
	W.O.D.:	rps/rnds/lps	HrMx%
1			
2			
3			
4			
5			
6			
7			
8			
9			
10			
11			
12			
		A.L.O.I @:	

Ana/Vo2 CARDIO INTERVALS

(Hvi's) mcw est. '13

	Date:	am or pm	Intervals:
	W.O.D.:	rps/rnds/lps	HrMx%
1			
2			
3			
4			
5			
6			
7			
8			
9			
10			
11			
12			
		A.L.O.I @:	

Ana/Vo2 CARDIO INTERVALS

(Hvi's) mcw est. '13

	Date:	am or pm	Intervals:
	W.O.D.:	rps/rnds/lps	HrMx%
1			
2			
3			
4			
5			
6			
7			
8			
9			
10			
11			
12			
		A.L.O.I @:	

Ana/Vo2 CARDIO INTERVALS
(Hvi's) mcw est. '13

	Date:	am or pm	Intervals:
	W.O.D.:	rps/rnds/lps	HrMx%
1			
2			
3			
4			
5			
6			
7			
8			
9			
10			
11			
12			
		A.L.O.I @:	

Ana/Vo2 CARDIO INTERVALS
(Hvi's) mcw est. '13

	Date:	am or pm	Intervals:
	W.O.D.:	rps/rnds/lps	HrMx%
1			
2			
3			
4			
5			
6			
7			
8			
9			
10			
11			
12			
		A.L.O.I @:	

Ana/Vo2 CARDIO INTERVALS
(Hvi's) mcw est. '13

	Date:	am or pm	Intervals:
	W.O.D.:	rps/rnds/lps	HrMx%
1			
2			
3			
4			
5			
6			
7			
8			
9			
10			
11			
12			
		A.L.O.I @:	

Ana/Vo2 CARDIO INTERVALS
(Hvi's) mcw est. '13

	Date:	am or pm	Intervals:
	W.O.D.:	rps/rnds/lps	HrMx%
1			
2			
3			
4			
5			
6			
7			
8			
9			
10			
11			
12			
		A.L.O.I @:	

Ana/Vo2 CARDIO INTERVALS
(Hvi's) mcw est. '13

	Date:	am or pm	Intervals:
	W.O.D.:	rps/rnds/lps	HrMx%
1			
2			
3			
4			
5			
6			
7			
8			
9			
10			
11			
12			
		A.L.O.I @:	

Ana/Vo2 CARDIO INTERVALS
(Hvi's) mcw est. '13

	Date:	am or pm	Intervals:
	W.O.D.:	rps/rnds/lps	HrMx%
1			
2			
3			
4			
5			
6			
7			
8			
9			
10			
11			
12			
		A.L.O.I @:	

Ana/Vo2 CARDIO INTERVALS
(Hvi's) mcw est. '13

	Date:	am or pm	Intervals:
	W.O.D.:	rps/rnds/lps	HrMx%
1			
2			
3			
4			
5			
6			
7			
8			
9			
10			
11			
12			
		A.L.O.I @:	

Ana/Vo2 CARDIO INTERVALS
(Hvi's) mcw est. '13

	Date:	am or pm	Intervals:
	W.O.D.:	rps/rnds/lps	HrMx%
1			
2			
3			
4			
5			
6			
7			
8			
9			
10			
11			
12			
		A.L.O.I @:	

Ana/Vo2 CARDIO INTERVALS
(Hvi's) mcw est. '13

	Date:	am or pm	Intervals:
	W.O.D.:	rps/rnds/lps	HrMx%
1			
2			
3			
4			
5			
6			
7			
8			
9			
10			
11			
12			
		A.L.O.I @:	

Ana/Vo2 CARDIO INTERVALS
(Hvi's) mcw est. '13

	Date:	am or pm	Intervals:
	W.O.D.:	rps/rnds/lps	HrMx%
1			
2			
3			
4			
5			
6			
7			
8			
9			
10			
11			
12			
		A.L.O.I @:	

Ana/Vo2 CARDIO INTERVALS
(Hvi's) mcw est. '13

	Date:	am or pm	Intervals:
	W.O.D.:	rps/rnds/lps	HrMx%
1			
2			
3			
4			
5			
6			
7			
8			
9			
10			
11			
12			
		A.L.O.I @:	

Ana/Vo2 CARDIO INTERVALS
(Hvi's) mcw est. '13

	Date:	am or pm	Intervals:
	W.O.D.:	rps/rnds/lps	HrMx%
1			
2			
3			
4			
5			
6			
7			
8			
9			
10			
11			
12			
		A.L.O.I @:	

Ana/Vo2 CARDIO INTERVALS
(Hvi's) mcw est. '13

	Date:	am or pm	Intervals:
	W.O.D.:	rps/rnds/lps	HrMx%
1			
2			
3			
4			
5			
6			
7			
8			
9			
10			
11			
12			
		A.L.O.I @:	

Ana/Vo2 CARDIO INTERVALS
(Hvi's) mcw est. '13

	Date:	am or pm	Intervals:
	W.O.D.:	rps/rnds/lps	HrMx%
1			
2			
3			
4			
5			
6			
7			
8			
9			
10			
11			
12			
		A.L.O.I @:	

Ana/Vo2 CARDIO INTERVALS
(Hvi's) mcw est. '13

	Date:	am or pm	Intervals:
	W.O.D.:	rps/rnds/lps	HrMx%
1			
2			
3			
4			
5			
6			
7			
8			
9			
10			
11			
12			
		A.L.O.I @:	

Ana/Vo2 CARDIO INTERVALS
(Hvi's) mcw est. '13

	Date:	am or pm	Intervals:
	W.O.D.:	rps/rnds/lps	HrMx%
1			
2			
3			
4			
5			
6			
7			
8			
9			
10			
11			
12			
		A.L.O.I @:	

Ana/Vo2 CARDIO INTERVALS
(Hvi's) mcw est. '13

	Date:	am or pm	Intervals:
	W.O.D.:	rps/rnds/lps	HrMx%
1			
2			
3			
4			
5			
6			
7			
8			
9			
10			
11			
12			
		A.L.O.I @:	

Ana/Vo2 CARDIO INTERVALS
(Hvi's) mcw est. '13

	Date:	am or pm	Intervals:
	W.O.D.:	rps/rnds/lps	HrMx%
1			
2			
3			
4			
5			
6			
7			
8			
9			
10			
11			
12			
		A.L.O.I @:	

Ana/Vo2 CARDIO INTERVALS

(Hvi's) mcw est. '13

	Date:	am or pm	Intervals:
	W.O.D.:	rps/rnds/lps	HrMx%
1			
2			
3			
4			
5			
6			
7			
8			
9			
10			
11			
12			
		A.L.O.I @:	

Ana/Vo2 CARDIO INTERVALS

(Hvi's) mcw est. '13

	Date:	am or pm	Intervals:
	W.O.D.:	rps/rnds/lps	HrMx%
1			
2			
3			
4			
5			
6			
7			
8			
9			
10			
11			
12			
		A.L.O.I @:	

Ana/Vo2 CARDIO INTERVALS

(Hvi's) mcw est. '13

	Date:	am or pm	Intervals:
	W.O.D.:	rps/rnds/lps	HrMx%
1			
2			
3			
4			
5			
6			
7			
8			
9			
10			
11			
12			
		A.L.O.I @:	

Ana/Vo2 CARDIO INTERVALS

(Hvi's) mcw est. '13

	Date:	am or pm	Intervals:
	W.O.D.:	rps/rnds/lps	HrMx%
1			
2			
3			
4			
5			
6			
7			
8			
9			
10			
11			
12			
		A.L.O.I @:	

Ana/Vo2 CARDIO INTERVALS

(Hvi's) mcw est. '13

	Date:	am or pm	Intervals:
	W.O.D.:	rps/rnds/lps	HrMx%
1			
2			
3			
4			
5			
6			
7			
8			
9			
10			
11			
12			
		A.L.O.I @:	

Ana/Vo2 CARDIO INTERVALS

(Hvi's) mcw est. '13

	Date:	am or pm	Intervals:
	W.O.D.:	rps/rnds/lps	HrMx%
1			
2			
3			
4			
5			
6			
7			
8			
9			
10			
11			
12			
		A.L.O.I @:	

FITNESS EVOLUTION NOTES:

Track your Training Effort Intensity Level Zones, Calorie Expense, and Personal Benchmark Record Data

DATE:__________ DATA:	DATE:__________ DATA:
DATE:__________ DATA:	DATE:__________ DATA:
DATE:__________ DATA:	DATE:__________ DATA:
DATE:__________ DATA:	DATE:__________ DATA:
DATE:__________ DATA:	DATE:__________ DATA:
DATE:__________ DATA:	DATE:__________ DATA:
DATE:__________ DATA:	DATE:__________ DATA:

FITNESS EVOLUTION NOTES:

Track your Training Effort Intensity Level Zones, Calorie Expense, and Personal Benchmark Record Data

DATE:________ DATA:	DATE:________ DATA:
DATE:________ DATA:	DATE:________ DATA:
DATE:________ DATA:	DATE:________ DATA:
DATE:________ DATA:	DATE:________ DATA:
DATE:________ DATA:	DATE:________ DATA:
DATE:________ DATA:	DATE:________ DATA:
DATE:________ DATA:	DATE:________ DATA:

NOTES:

NOTES:

6 Week Training Calendar
Month Year

SUNDAY	MONDAY	TUESDAY	WEDNESDAY	THURSDAY	FRIDAY	SATURDAY

Week 1

Date:	Date:	Date:	Date:	Date:	Date:	Date:
Mileage:	Mileage:	Mileage:	Mileage:	Mileage:	Mileage:	Mileage:

Week 2

Date:	Date:	Date:	Date:	Date:	Date:	Date:
Mileage:	Mileage:	Mileage:	Mileage:	Mileage:	Mileage:	Mileage:

Week 3

Date:	Date:	Date:	Date:	Date:	Date:	Date:
Mileage:	Mileage:	Mileage:	Mileage:	Mileage:	Mileage:	Mileage:

Week 4

Date:	Date:	Date:	Date:	Date:	Date:	Date:
Mileage:	Mileage:	Mileage:	Mileage:	Mileage:	Mileage:	Mileage:

Week 5

Date:	Date:	Date:	Date:	Date:	Date:	Date:
Mileage:	Mileage:	Mileage:	Mileage:	Mileage:	Mileage:	Mileage:

Week 6

Date:	Date:	Date:	Date:	Date:	Date:	Date:
Mileage:	Mileage:	Mileage:	Mileage:	Mileage:	Mileage:	Mileage:

Ana/Vo2 CARDIO INTERVALS
(Hvi's) mcw est. '13

	Date:	am or pm	Intervals:
	W.O.D.:	rps/rnds/lps	HrMx%
1			
2			
3			
4			
5			
6			
7			
8			
9			
10			
11			
12			
		A.L.O.I @:	

Ana/Vo2 CARDIO INTERVALS
(Hvi's) mcw est. '13

	Date:	am or pm	Intervals:
	W.O.D.:	rps/rnds/lps	HrMx%
1			
2			
3			
4			
5			
6			
7			
8			
9			
10			
11			
12			
		A.L.O.I @:	

Ana/Vo2 CARDIO INTERVALS
(Hvi's) mcw est. '13

	Date:	am or pm	Intervals:
	W.O.D.:	rps/rnds/lps	HrMx%
1			
2			
3			
4			
5			
6			
7			
8			
9			
10			
11			
12			
		A.L.O.I @:	

Ana/Vo2 CARDIO INTERVALS
(Hvi's) mcw est. '13

	Date:	am or pm	Intervals:
	W.O.D.:	rps/rnds/lps	HrMx%
1			
2			
3			
4			
5			
6			
7			
8			
9			
10			
11			
12			
		A.L.O.I @:	

Ana/Vo2 CARDIO INTERVALS
(Hvi's) mcw est. '13

	Date:	am or pm	Intervals:
	W.O.D.:	rps/rnds/lps	HrMx%
1			
2			
3			
4			
5			
6			
7			
8			
9			
10			
11			
12			
		A.L.O.I @:	

Ana/Vo2 CARDIO INTERVALS
(Hvi's) mcw est. '13

	Date:	am or pm	Intervals:
	W.O.D.:	rps/rnds/lps	HrMx%
1			
2			
3			
4			
5			
6			
7			
8			
9			
10			
11			
12			
		A.L.O.I @:	

Ana/Vo2 CARDIO INTERVALS

(Hvi's) mcw est. '13

	Date:	am or pm	Intervals:
	W.O.D.:	rps/rnds/lps	HrMx%
1			
2			
3			
4			
5			
6			
7			
8			
9			
10			
11			
12			
		A.L.O.I @:	

Ana/Vo2 CARDIO INTERVALS

(Hvi's) mcw est. '13

	Date:	am or pm	Intervals:
	W.O.D.:	rps/rnds/lps	HrMx%
1			
2			
3			
4			
5			
6			
7			
8			
9			
10			
11			
12			
		A.L.O.I @:	

Ana/Vo2 CARDIO INTERVALS

(Hvi's) mcw est. '13

	Date:	am or pm	Intervals:
	W.O.D.:	rps/rnds/lps	HrMx%
1			
2			
3			
4			
5			
6			
7			
8			
9			
10			
11			
12			
		A.L.O.I @:	

Ana/Vo2 CARDIO INTERVALS

(Hvi's) mcw est. '13

	Date:	am or pm	Intervals:
	W.O.D.:	rps/rnds/lps	HrMx%
1			
2			
3			
4			
5			
6			
7			
8			
9			
10			
11			
12			
		A.L.O.I @:	

Ana/Vo2 CARDIO INTERVALS

(Hvi's) mcw est. '13

	Date:	am or pm	Intervals:
	W.O.D.:	rps/rnds/lps	HrMx%
1			
2			
3			
4			
5			
6			
7			
8			
9			
10			
11			
12			
		A.L.O.I @:	

Ana/Vo2 CARDIO INTERVALS

(Hvi's) mcw est. '13

	Date:	am or pm	Intervals:
	W.O.D.:	rps/rnds/lps	HrMx%
1			
2			
3			
4			
5			
6			
7			
8			
9			
10			
11			
12			
		A.L.O.I @:	

Ana/Vo2 CARDIO INTERVALS

(Hvi's) mcw est. '13

	Date:	am or pm	Intervals:
	W.O.D.:	rps/rnds/lps	HrMx%
1			
2			
3			
4			
5			
6			
7			
8			
9			
10			
11			
12			
		A.L.O.I @:	

Ana/Vo2 CARDIO INTERVALS

(Hvi's) mcw est. '13

	Date:	am or pm	Intervals:
	W.O.D.:	rps/rnds/lps	HrMx%
1			
2			
3			
4			
5			
6			
7			
8			
9			
10			
11			
12			
		A.L.O.I @:	

Ana/Vo2 CARDIO INTERVALS

(Hvi's) mcw est. '13

	Date:	am or pm	Intervals:
	W.O.D.:	rps/rnds/lps	HrMx%
1			
2			
3			
4			
5			
6			
7			
8			
9			
10			
11			
12			
		A.L.O.I @:	

Ana/Vo2 CARDIO INTERVALS

(Hvi's) mcw est. '13

	Date:	am or pm	Intervals:
	W.O.D.:	rps/rnds/lps	HrMx%
1			
2			
3			
4			
5			
6			
7			
8			
9			
10			
11			
12			
		A.L.O.I @:	

Ana/Vo2 CARDIO INTERVALS

(Hvi's) mcw est. '13

	Date:	am or pm	Intervals:
	W.O.D.:	rps/rnds/lps	HrMx%
1			
2			
3			
4			
5			
6			
7			
8			
9			
10			
11			
12			
		A.L.O.I @:	

Ana/Vo2 CARDIO INTERVALS

(Hvi's) mcw est. '13

	Date:	am or pm	Intervals:
	W.O.D.:	rps/rnds/lps	HrMx%
1			
2			
3			
4			
5			
6			
7			
8			
9			
10			
11			
12			
		A.L.O.I @:	

Ana/Vo2 CARDIO INTERVALS

(Hvi's) mcw est. '13

	Date:	am or pm	Intervals:
	W.O.D.:	rps/rnds/lps	HrMx%
1			
2			
3			
4			
5			
6			
7			
8			
9			
10			
11			
12			
		A.L.O.I @:	

Ana/Vo2 CARDIO INTERVALS

(Hvi's) mcw est. '13

	Date:	am or pm	Intervals:
	W.O.D.:	rps/rnds/lps	HrMx%
1			
2			
3			
4			
5			
6			
7			
8			
9			
10			
11			
12			
		A.L.O.I @:	

Ana/Vo2 CARDIO INTERVALS

(Hvi's) mcw est. '13

	Date:	am or pm	Intervals:
	W.O.D.:	rps/rnds/lps	HrMx%
1			
2			
3			
4			
5			
6			
7			
8			
9			
10			
11			
12			
		A.L.O.I @:	

Ana/Vo2 CARDIO INTERVALS

(Hvi's) mcw est. '13

	Date:	am or pm	Intervals:
	W.O.D.:	rps/rnds/lps	HrMx%
1			
2			
3			
4			
5			
6			
7			
8			
9			
10			
11			
12			
		A.L.O.I @:	

Ana/Vo2 CARDIO INTERVALS

(Hvi's) mcw est. '13

	Date:	am or pm	Intervals:
	W.O.D.:	rps/rnds/lps	HrMx%
1			
2			
3			
4			
5			
6			
7			
8			
9			
10			
11			
12			
		A.L.O.I @:	

Ana/Vo2 CARDIO INTERVALS

(Hvi's) mcw est. '13

	Date:	am or pm	Intervals:
	W.O.D.:	rps/rnds/lps	HrMx%
1			
2			
3			
4			
5			
6			
7			
8			
9			
10			
11			
12			
		A.L.O.I @:	

Ana/Vo2 CARDIO INTERVALS

(Hvi's) mcw est. '13

	Date:	am or pm	Intervals:
	W.O.D.:	rps/rnds/lps	HrMx%
1			
2			
3			
4			
5			
6			
7			
8			
9			
10			
11			
12			
		A.L.O.I @:	

Ana/Vo2 CARDIO INTERVALS

(Hvi's) mcw est. '13

	Date:	am or pm	Intervals:
	W.O.D.:	rps/rnds/lps	HrMx%
1			
2			
3			
4			
5			
6			
7			
8			
9			
10			
11			
12			
		A.L.O.I @:	

Ana/Vo2 CARDIO INTERVALS

(Hvi's) mcw est. '13

	Date:	am or pm	Intervals:
	W.O.D.:	rps/rnds/lps	HrMx%
1			
2			
3			
4			
5			
6			
7			
8			
9			
10			
11			
12			
		A.L.O.I @:	

Ana/Vo2 CARDIO INTERVALS

(Hvi's) mcw est. '13

	Date:	am or pm	Intervals:
	W.O.D.:	rps/rnds/lps	HrMx%
1			
2			
3			
4			
5			
6			
7			
8			
9			
10			
11			
12			
		A.L.O.I @:	

Ana/Vo2 CARDIO INTERVALS

(Hvi's) mcw est. '13

	Date:	am or pm	Intervals:
	W.O.D.:	rps/rnds/lps	HrMx%
1			
2			
3			
4			
5			
6			
7			
8			
9			
10			
11			
12			
		A.L.O.I @:	

Ana/Vo2 CARDIO INTERVALS

(Hvi's) mcw est. '13

	Date:	am or pm	Intervals:
	W.O.D.:	rps/rnds/lps	HrMx%
1			
2			
3			
4			
5			
6			
7			
8			
9			
10			
11			
12			
		A.L.O.I @:	

FITNESS EVOLUTION NOTES:

Track your Training Effort Intensity Level Zones, Calorie Expense, and Personal Benchmark Record Data

DATE:__________ DATA:	DATE:__________ DATA:
DATE:__________ DATA:	DATE:__________ DATA:
DATE:__________ DATA:	DATE:__________ DATA:
DATE:__________ DATA:	DATE:__________ DATA:
DATE:__________ DATA:	DATE:__________ DATA:
DATE:__________ DATA:	DATE:__________ DATA:
DATE:__________ DATA:	DATE:__________ DATA:

FITNESS EVOLUTION NOTES:

Track your Training Effort Intensity Level Zones, Calorie Expense, and Personal Benchmark Record Data

DATE:__________ DATA:	DATE:__________ DATA:
DATE:__________ DATA:	DATE:__________ DATA:
DATE:__________ DATA:	DATE:__________ DATA:
DATE:__________ DATA:	DATE:__________ DATA:
DATE:__________ DATA:	DATE:__________ DATA:
DATE:__________ DATA:	DATE:__________ DATA:
DATE:__________ DATA:	DATE:__________ DATA:

NOTES:

NOTES:

Note From the Author

This 1-Year Calendar Training Journal was created to be a Supplement to the Original Copyrighted Version of The Science Within A Heathen Warriors Fitness Manual.

Features within:

- A Portable log book made easier to transport to the gym or any recreation area
- It can be used with the Original Manual and/or personal exercise program
- eBook readers and all Athletes
- 1-Year Calendar Log
- 7 Av²/ci WOD sheets per six-week Calendar
- Progress Notes for Documenting your Fitness Evolution
- Blank Lined Paper for your writing needs
- Portable reference charts found in Original Manual Section Five
- 5k & 10k 6-week Training plans found in Original Manual Section Five

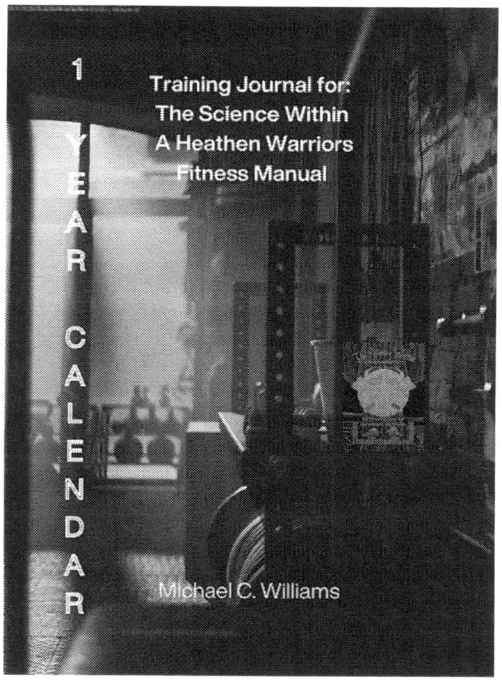
1 YEAR CALENDAR
Training Journal for:
The Science Within
A Heathen Warriors
Fitness Manual
Michael C. Williams

Made in the USA
Coppell, TX
08 February 2024

28788841R00190